5TH Edition

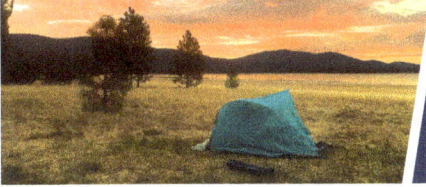

BEST TENT
Camping

Northern
CALIFORNIA

YOUR CAR-CAMPING GUIDE TO SCENIC BEAUTY, THE SOUNDS
OF NATURE, AND AN ESCAPE FROM CIVILIZATION

Best Tent Camping: Northern California

Published by Menasha Ridge Press
Distributed by Publishers Group West

Library of Congress Cataloging-in-Publication Data

Names: Speicher, Wendy, 1979- author.
Title: Best tent camping. Northern California : your car-camping guide to scenic beauty, the sounds of nature, and
    an escape from civilization / Wendy Speicher.
Description: Fifth Edition. | Birmingham, Alabama : Menasha Ridge Press, your guide to the outdoors since 1982,
    [2017] | "Distributed by Publishers Group West"—T.p. verso. | Includes index.
Identifiers: LCCN 2017015731 | ISBN 9781634040440 (paperback : alk. paper) | ISBN 9781634040457 (ebook) |
    ISBN 9781634041966 (hardcover)
Subjects: LCSH: Camp sites, facilities, etc.—California, Northern—Directories. | Camping—California, Northern--
    Guidebooks. | California, Northern—Guidebooks.
Classification: LCC GV191.42.C2 S64 2017 | DDC 796.5409794—dc23
LC record available at https://lccn.loc.gov/2017015731

Cover and text design by Jon Norberg
Cover photos by Wendy Speicher
Maps by Steve Jones
Photos: Shutterstock (pages 14, 15, 19, 30, 33, 39, 40, 51, 78, 81, 107, 111, 135, and 169). All others by Wendy Speicher
    unless otherwise noted on page.
Project editor: Kate Johnson
Proofreader: Rebecca Henderson
Indexer: Rich Carlson

MENASHA RIDGE PRESS
An imprint of AdventureKEEN
2204 First Ave. S., Ste. 102
Birmingham, AL 35233

Visit menasharidge.com for a complete listing of our books and for ordering information. Contact us at our website, at
facebook.com/menasharidge, or at twitter.com/menasharidge with questions or comments. To find out more about
who we are and what we're doing, visit blog.menasharidge.com.

Front cover: Merrill Campground (top; see page 91) and Middle Falls at Fowlers Campground (see page 101)

5TH Edition

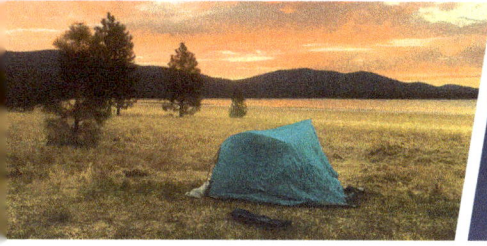

BEST TENT
Camping

Northern
CALIFORNIA

YOUR CAR-CAMPING GUIDE TO SCENIC BEAUTY, THE SOUNDS
OF NATURE, AND AN ESCAPE FROM CIVILIZATION

Wendy Speicher

MENASHA RIDGE PRESS
Your Guide to the Outdoors Since 1982

Northern California Campground Locator Map

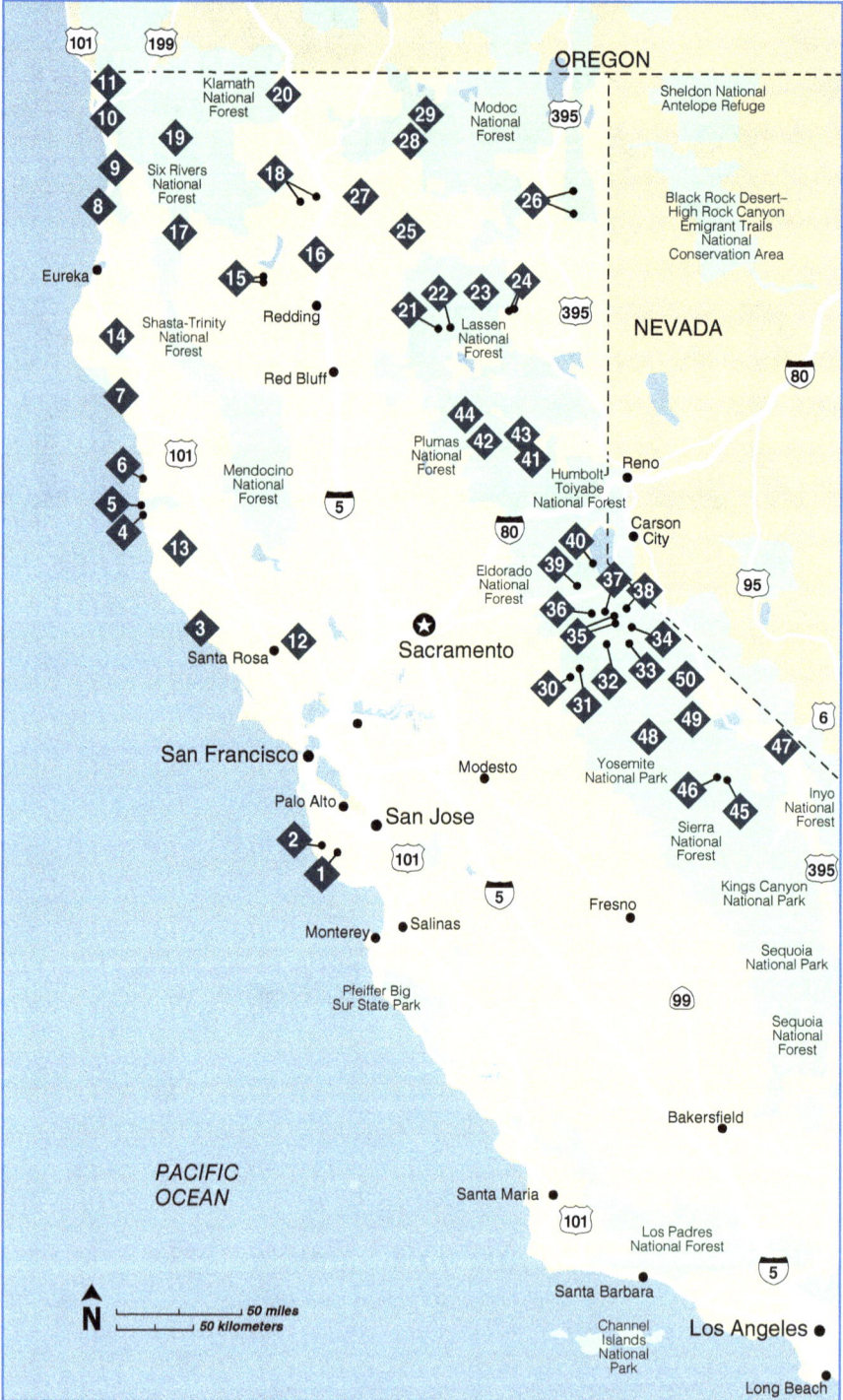

101 199

OREGON

Klamath National Forest

Modoc National Forest 395

Sheldon National Antelope Refuge

NEVADA

Six Rivers National Forest

Black Rock Desert–High Rock Canyon Emigrant Trails National Conservation Area

Eureka

Shasta-Trinity National Forest

Redding

Red Bluff

Lassen National Forest

395

80

Plumas National Forest

Reno

Humbolt Toiyabe National Forest

101

Mendocino National Forest

5

80

Carson City

Eldorado National Forest

95

Santa Rosa

12

Sacramento

6

San Francisco

Modesto

Yosemite National Park

Inyo National Forest

47

Palo Alto

San Jose

Sierra National Forest

395

101

5

Fresno

Kings Canyon National Park

Monterey Salinas

Sequoia National Park

Pfeiffer Big Sur State Park

99

Sequoia National Forest

Bakersfield

PACIFIC OCEAN

Santa Maria

101

Los Padres National Forest

5

Santa Barbara

N
50 miles
50 kilometers

Channel Islands National Park

Los Angeles

Long Beach

CONTENTS

THE CASCADE RANGE 81

THE SIERRA NEVADA 110

YOSEMITE 156

Map Legend

N (North indicator)	← (Off-map or pinpoint-indication arrow)	15A 37 H host 10 5 (Individual tent sites, cabins, and RV sites)	Group camping sites/areas
Sacramento ✪ Capital	**Azalea** ● City or town	**NATIONAL FOREST** **STATE PARK** **WILDLIFE REFUGE** — Public lands	Hiking and biking trails
5 Interstate highways	101 89 US highways	1 236 State roads	Maple Grove Rd. Other roads
Dirt/gravel road	Boardwalk	Opal Creek River or stream	Juniper Lake Lake or pond

Amphitheater		Gate		RV parking
Basketball court		Group campsite		Sheltered area
Bridge		Horseshoe pit		Sheltered picnic area
Boat ramp		Information		Showers
Campfire		Laundry		Store
Campground		Parking		Stock corral
Concession/ food stand		Pet walking area		Swimming area
Dining		Phone access		Trash disposal
Dump station		Picnic area		Volleyball
Firewood		Point of interest		Water access
Fishing		Ranger station/office		Waterfall
		Restroom		Wheelchair access

ACKNOWLEDGMENTS

It literally takes a village to create a book, and in that spirit I have a lot of people to thank! First, the friendly, encouraging, and incredibly patient people at AdventureKEEN, who have put so much time, energy, and love into this book. Thank you to my acquisition editor, Tim Jackson, for believing in me and keeping me going; to Amber Henderson for your patience, insight, and attention to all the nitty-gritty details; to Kate Johnson for helping us bring this project over the finish line; and to the cartographers and designers who put together the often handwritten notes and pictures into a beautiful compilation. I am deeply grateful.

Next, I owe so much to the initial authors of this book—Bill Mai and later Cindy Coloma. I was fortunate to simply build off of their in-depth research and spot-on recommendations. It was a great pleasure to revisit and discover many of these stellar sites and find that not much had changed from when they originally selected these areas as Northern California's best. Thank you so much to both of you for setting an enjoyable, easy to read, and informational tone that will continue to be the legacy of this title.

It also takes a village to run a campground, and so I'd like to thank all of the campground staff who manage, protect, and care for these beautiful places so everyone can enjoy their stay. And also, to each and every ranger and host who took the time to answer all of my questions, help with on-the-ground research, and respond to my many e-mails and phone calls. Without your help and local expertise, this book literally would not have been possible.

Revising a book of this magnitude with so much field work takes a supportive family, and I am grateful for mine. I'll start with my dad, a lifelong fan, who not only instilled in me a deep appreciation of adventure, time spent outdoors, and camping at an early age but also took off 10 days to join my 4-year-old son, Archer, and I on a whirlwind trip into Northern California's Cascade Range to research new entries and revisit old sites. Dad's attention to detail and playful, easygoing attitude made the week extremely productive and an experience my son and I will hold dear forever. I also want to thank my husband's parents, Bob and Grace Speicher, who joined me on a couple of fun trips researching new sites as well and provided recommendations for others. Every trip with the Speichers is always characterized by making new friends with the site neighbors and enjoying the outdoors in ultimate style.

Last, but definitely not least, I must thank my husband, Greg Speicher, and my son, Archer. Greg's support and willingness to rearrange his busy work schedule to accommodate my need to get boots on the ground either with the family or on my own was critical in my ability to finish this book. And Archer's easygoing, curious, and outdoorsy nature made each adventure that much more memorable. There is literally nothing like sharing the joy of camping and nature with a child, and this helped motivate my research so other families can enjoy their explorations of Northern California as much as we have.

From the bottom of my heart,
Wendy Speicher

PREFACE

What a time to be alive! When armed with our various technological devices, our access to information is fluid and faster than ever before. For many of us, the day begins with our phone alarm clock that may even greet us with an up-to-date report on the quality of our sleep the night before. We scroll our various media feeds while the coffee gets hot and leave the house with a preloaded map set on navigation, complete with directions, estimated arrival times, and suggested detours based on traffic patterns. Our phones guide us step by step to our destination, often determined by scouring Yelp and Google reviews, while we stream music from our favorite station and our daughter checks social media in the passenger seat.

Sound familiar? To say that we are the generation of "plugged in" is hardly a stretch for many of us, especially those who are currently living in Northern California. But to say that there is an insatiable desire for more than what our screens offer us is, again, hardly a stretch. And while most of us feel the drain of such constant device interaction, others embrace these times as an opportunity to explore new freedoms—some managing online businesses from their campsites or even working remotely from the trail in many cases.

Whatever "camp" you find yourself in, most of us expect real-time information and updates. That type of accuracy is impossible to achieve when writing a book. Budgets get cut, storms wash out roads, and businesses close. For real-time answers, please use the websites we have listed in this book, or call ahead to make sure you don't run into any snags.

Enjoy stunning views and whale-watching from the steep cliffs at Patrick's Point State Park, one of Northern California's most scenic (see page 39).

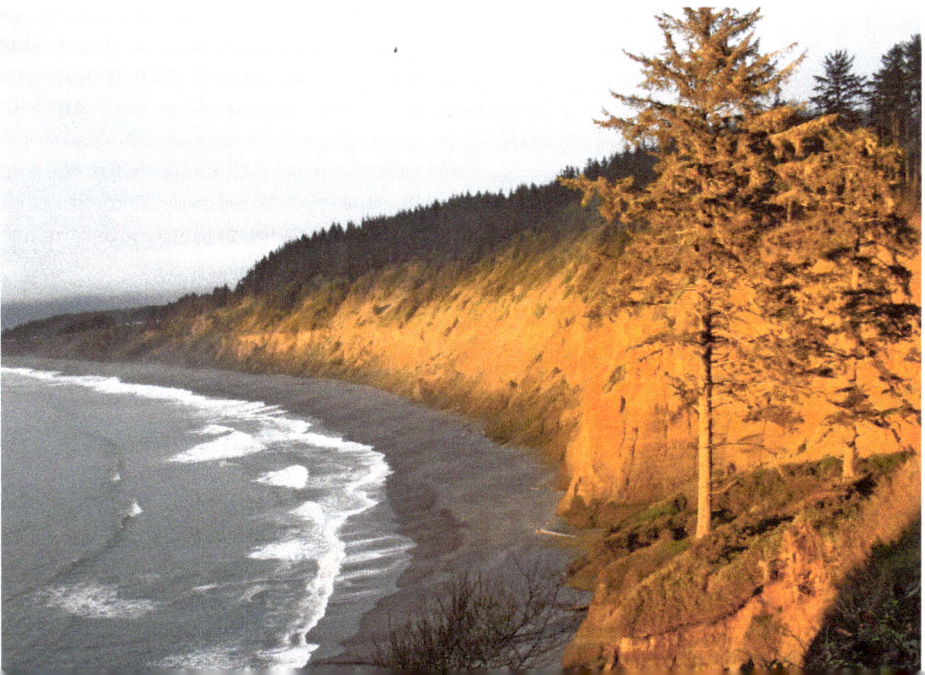

photographed by Saylor Moss

This book is intended to help you design an outdoor camping experience that nourishes your human need for natural connection. It is intended to inspire you to explore new places—or discover old ones with renewed perspective—and to seek new adventures, all while giving you the tools to make these new dreams a reality. Study these pages and you'll find out where, why, when, and how to go, and what to do once you get there. But that will just be the beginning, as your presence and participation will make the experience uniquely yours.

We've selected 50 of the best campgrounds in six regions of Northern California. The diversity in elevation, geography, size, and amenities is unparalleled. This guide is organized from south to north and west to east, to make planning a trip that fits into your schedule easy. It also assists you in planning a trip that incorporates any additional interests that draw you into the woods, such as mountain biking, rock climbing, birding, surfing, sipping fine wines, soaking in natural hot springs, or simply unplugging. In an age where we are increasingly attaining new technological advances, this book presents an opportunity to reconnect with the natural environment while maintaining many of the comforts of home. Tent camping offers us the opportunity to inhale what may be the most potent medicine of our time: a simple night of fresh air.

I moved to Northern California at the turn of this century. Wide-eyed and eager to explore, I made my initial home in the Yosemite Valley as a summer employee, in service to the throngs of people who don't look where they are walking because their eyes are glued to the valley's impressive granite walls. In my free time, I went off the beaten path, hiked, rock climbed, and learned to whitewater kayak. I took those skills on the road, landing next in the Lake Tahoe area to pursue the lucrative lifestyle of ski bum then enrolling in college to study journalism and geography in the redwoods at Humboldt State University. I've always said that I'm all about my wallpaper: I live where it's pretty outside because that's where I like to be. For me and for this reason, camping is a natural fit. I camp because I am a sucker for luxury, the kind of luxury that means I can have front-door access to jaw-dropping views and back-door access to superb recreation, all on a shoestring budget that maintains my freedom. As a Michigan native, my impression of the California experience is "only the best," and to that mantra I say, "amen."

So where do you want to go? What kinds of activities do you prefer? Are you seeking high mountains with hot showers or a lake view au naturel? There's a campground and region to fit every interest and to satisfy every outdoor dream; you can fill your trip with activities or keep it relaxing and low-key.

And yet, even with a guidebook, we can never predict what we'll find, or what will find us, until we venture out. Whatever happens, we'll take the experiences back to our cities and towns and civilized lives. And we'll plan for the next trip. Because this is why we love camping.

—Wendy Speicher

BEST CAMPGROUNDS

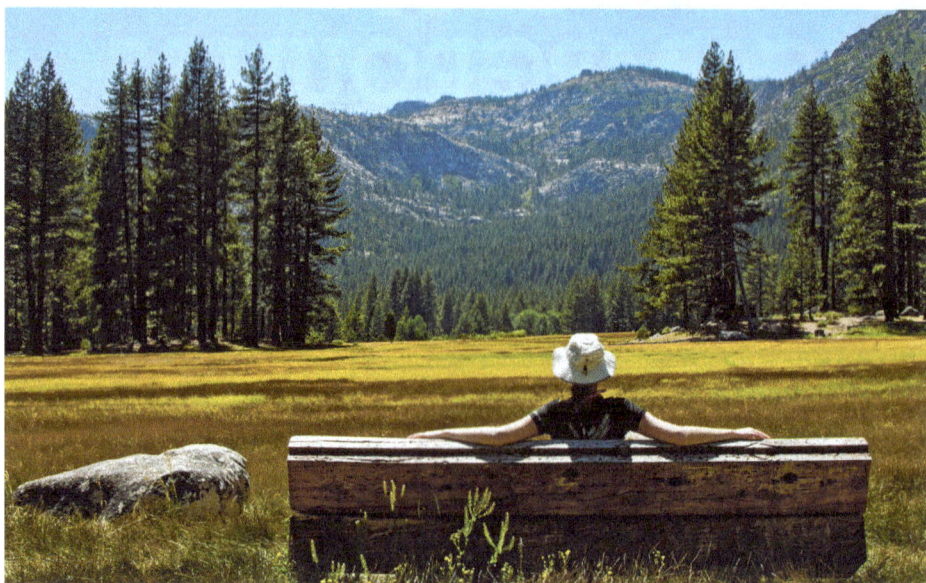

Grover Hot Springs State Park offers year-round camping with access to hot springs in the stunning Sierra Nevada *(see page 135)*.

BEST FOR FISHING AND BOATING

BEST FOR HIKING

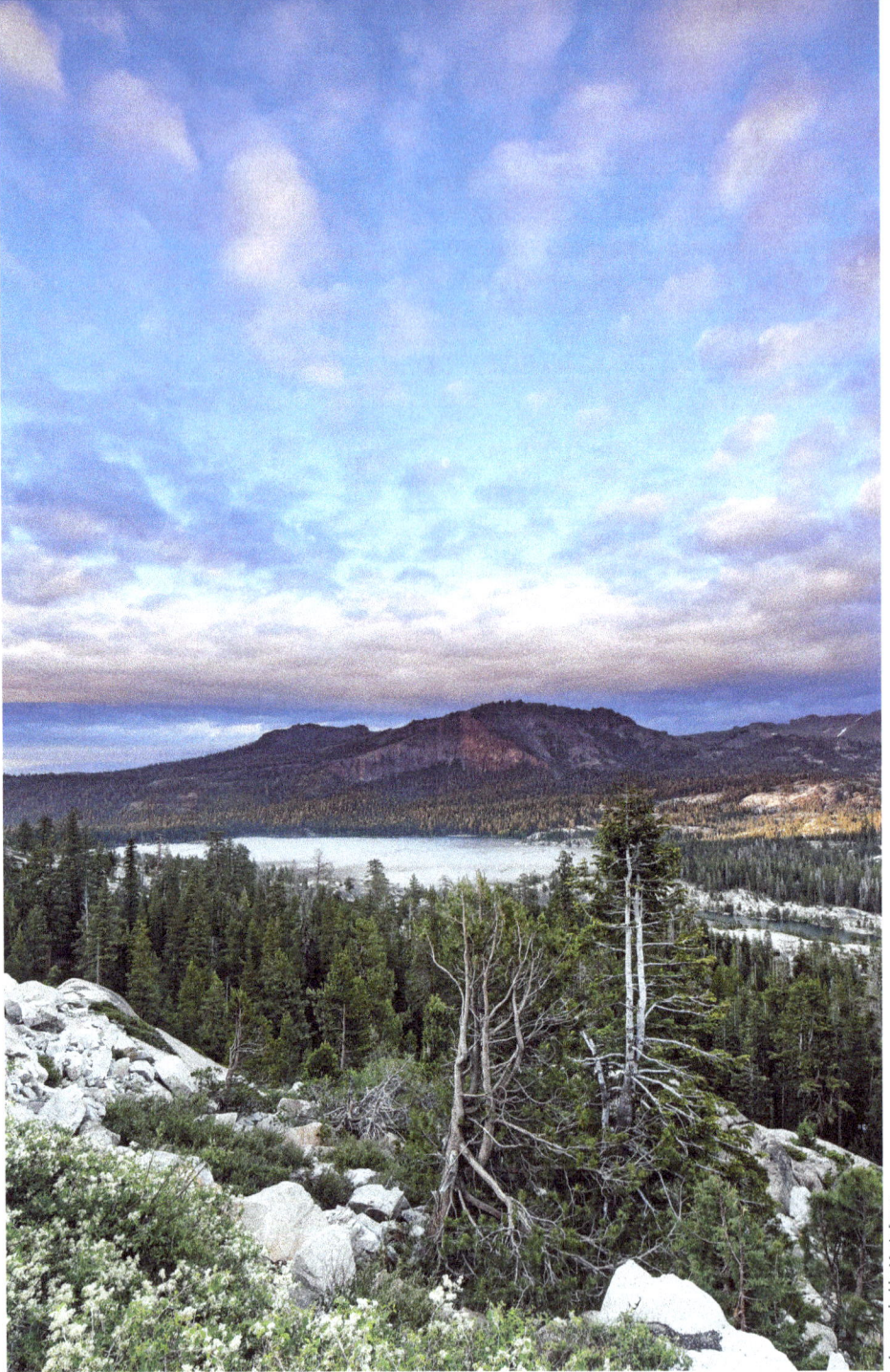

Silver Lake East Campground offers plenty of high mountain lake exploration on the Carson Pass *(see page 129)*.

photographed by Mario Lopez

INTRODUCTION

A WORD ABOUT THIS BOOK AND NORTHERN CALIFORNIA TENT CAMPING

Camp Northern California. Drive up I-5 and feel the big granite block of the Sierra Nevada looming to the east, 400 miles long. Ahead, in the Shasta-Trinity, is Mount Shasta, 14,161 feet high and topped with snow. To the west are the rolling hills of the Wine Country and the Coast Range, an ocean of sharp mountains and redwoods dipping down into the Pacific, where the white-blue waves break on rocky shores. From Lassen Volcanic National Park north, the Cascade Range is all volcanic, up past Alturas to Lava Beds National Monument. The weather is as wild as the land. Nowhere else can you feel so remote, camp on such wild, beautiful land, and fish untamed rivers running to the sea.

THE RATINGS AND RATING CATEGORIES

Evaluating campgrounds requires some finesse, and in the end it is more of an art than a science. For a quick summary of what qualities make these campgrounds worth visiting, each is rated on six attributes—beauty, privacy, spaciousness, quiet, security, and cleanliness. A five-star scale is used—five stars is best, and one star is acceptable. Not every campground in this book can pull a high score in every category. Sometimes a very worthwhile campground is located on terrain that makes it difficult to provide a lot of space, for example. In these cases, high marks in beauty or quiet may trump room to stretch out. In any case, the star-rating system is a handy tool to help you pinpoint the campground that will fit your personal requirements.

★★★★★   The site is **ideal** in that category.

★★★★   The site is **exemplary** in that category.

★★★   The site is **very good** in that category.

★★   The site is **above average** in that category.

★   The site is **acceptable** in that category.

BEAUTY

Though all 50 campgrounds in this book are beautiful, some are absolutely sensational, and these rate five stars. Mountains, streams, waterfalls, and sunsets all conspire for a drop-dead campground personality. One- to four-star campgrounds are not poor, either, but possess a less spectacular beauty that will grow on you.

PRIVACY

Some campgrounds are beautifully built. The sites are arranged to take maximum advantage of the contour of the land, and the vegetation gives each one the most privacy possible. Good architecture cuts down on the cringe factor when other campers pull in next door. A bit of privacy makes you feel at home from the moment you step out of your car. What a difference!

SPACIOUSNESS

I want flat land to pitch a tent on. And I want the flat area far enough from the picnic table so my camping mate can make coffee without waking me, and far enough from the fire pit that the embers don't burn little holes in the tent. And I want a view. A view from each campsite is part of the spacious feeling that qualifies a campground for five stars in this category.

QUIET

Quiet is part of beautiful. There's nothing like the sound of a generator or a boom box to ruin a beautiful campsite. I consider white noise such as the roar of a river to raise the quiet rating, since it is a natural noise and drowns out the sounds of other campers.

SECURITY

Most of the campsites in the top 50 have campground hosts that keep a good eye on the property, which makes the campground safer than a good neighborhood. The farther the campground is from an urban center, the more secure it is. Often, you can leave your valuables with the hosts if you're going to be gone for a day or so, but don't leave little things lying around. A blue jay will take off with a pair of sunglasses, and you never can tell what a visiting bear will decide has food value.

CLEANLINESS

Most campgrounds in the top 50 are well tended. Sometimes, on big weekends, places can get a little rank—not unlike one's kitchen after a big party. I appreciate the little things, like the campground host who came around with a rake after each site was vacated to police the place. That particular campground received five stars in the cleanliness department.

THE OVERVIEW MAP AND MAP LEGEND

Use the overview map on page iv to pinpoint the location of each campground. Each campground's number follows it throughout this guidebook, from the overview map to the table of contents to the profile's first page. A map legend that details the symbols found on the campground-layout maps appears on page vii.

CAMPGROUND-LAYOUT MAPS

Each profile contains a detailed map of campground sites, internal roads, facilities, and other key items.

CAMPGROUND ENTRANCE GPS COORDINATES

Each of the 50 profiles in this guidebook includes the GPS coordinates for that site's entrance. The intersection of the latitude (north) and longitude (west) coordinates orient you at the entrance. Please note that this guidebook uses the degree–decimal minute format for presenting the GPS coordinates. Example:

N37° 10.338′ W122° 13.320′

To convert GPS coordinates from degrees, minutes, and seconds to the above degree–decimal minute format, the seconds are divided by 60. For more on GPS technology, visit usgs.gov.

GEOGRAPHY

For the purposes of this book, Northern California is everything above a line drawn from Santa Cruz across to Yosemite National Park and the Nevada border and north to the Oregon border. This area is divided into the Coast Range, Wine Country, the Cascade Range, the Sierra Nevada, Yosemite, and Shasta-Trinity.

The Coast Range includes the hundreds of miles of rock cliffs, sandy coves, and beaches between Santa Cruz and Oregon, as well as the mountains running down to the sea. Wine Country is defined as the fertile hills and valleys that lie on the eastern side of the Coast Range. The Shasta-Trinity region of California extends from the top of the Sacramento Valley north to Oregon until it reaches a handshake toward the coastal ranges. East of I-5 is the Cascade Range in the north, the Modoc plateau, and Lassen Volcanic National Park, where the Cascade Range runs south and merges with the Sierra Nevada and then south into the wonderland that is Yosemite.

WHERE TO GO AND WHEN

Depending on elevation and location, great camping in Northern California can be found May–October, and even year-round. Camping in the mountains is mostly for late spring, summer, and early fall. The Sierra Nevada, Cascade, Yosemite, and Shasta-Trinity climate is fairly reliable as soon as the winter snowpack melts. But until summer fully arrives, watch the weather. It can get bone-cold in the higher regions even in the summer.

Summer heat (June–mid-September) can be sweltering at lower elevations, especially in the Cascades and Shasta-Trinity. This is the perfect time to spend the afternoons on the lake after a morning exploring waterfalls and caves. Or pack your gear and escape the heat at those high mountain campgrounds that can be enjoyed only a few months out of the year.

The coast can be explored anytime, but it's especially pleasant September–November, when there is less fog and more sunshine. The coastal climate is an inconsistent tyrant the rest of the year, but those sunshiny days quickly dry the memories of those filled with rain and fog. Enjoy the sun; it may be gone within hours or hang around for days—neither you nor the weatherman can guess which. Wine Country can also be enjoyed year-round but is often best in the spring and fall.

Some mountain campgrounds in Northern California are open even in the winter for the hardy breed who want to snow-camp. Watch the weather, come prepared, and let a few people know you're there—including a local ranger station.

WEATHER

In general, winters in Northern California are cool and wet, while summers are warm and dry. Beyond that general trend, summers on the coast tend to be cool and foggy, especially in the morning but sometimes all day, with June and July often hit the worst. Winters in the Sierra Nevada, Yosemite, and the Cascade Range are usually snowed in. Summers in the Shasta-Trinity and the Cascade Range tend to be hotter than those in the Sierra Nevada and in Yosemite, but in any mountainous area, expect hot, clear sunny days with the occasional afternoon thunderstorm and cool nights. Wine Country tends to be rainy in the winter and spring and usually just far enough inland to be out of reach of the summer fog. Expect hot summer temperatures.

ROADS AND VEHICLES

Road closures, summer construction crews, and traffic congestion are real issues along Northern California's highways. Before you go, check Caltrans (dot.ca.gov) to make sure the roads you intend to drive are indeed open. The regions most affected by seasonal closures are in the Sierra Nevada and Yosemite. CA 4 over Ebbetts Pass, CA 89 through Lassen, CA 108 over Sonora Pass, CA 120 over Tioga Pass through Yosemite, and CA 203 in Mammoth Lakes have historically been closed from early November through late June and early July with heavy winter snowfalls but can open as early as April and May.

In the wintertime, if you're planning any travel in or through mountainous regions, make sure that you either have four-wheel drive, all-wheel drive, and/or chains for your vehicle. Traffic patterns tend to follow the traditional workweek, with heaviest traffic away from metro areas on Friday evening and heaviest traffic heading toward metro areas on Sunday afternoon/evening. Plan your trip accordingly.

PERMITS AND ACCESS

The State of California sells a number of day-use passes to all of its state parks; these can be purchased online at parks.ca.gov or in person at any state park. The passes grant access for day use only and will not save you any money on camping reservations.

Most of California's national parks require a national park pass to enter. Passes can be purchased at the park entrance station or online. If you plan to visit a number of national parks and/or stay for more than seven days, purchasing the America the Beautiful Pass for $80 is a good way to go. Special discounts are available for veterans and seniors. Visit nps.gov for more details.

Some national forests require a backcountry permit to travel outside of the general campground area. Some parks and campgrounds require a special permit to have a fire. Please inquire about the restrictions and rules pertaining to your specific area when you check into your campsite.

GOOD PLANNING

A little planning makes a good camping trip great, and, honestly, in many cases it's best to look six or seven months ahead. First decide where and when you want to go. Most of California's state parks are at least partly on the reservation system. Especially if your plan includes a weekend, mark your calendar for seven months before your intended trip (six months for national parks), and set your alarm for 8 a.m. Plan to get online and make a reservation. Northern California is a popular place to camp, and a lot of people are in on the secret. Plan early and you'll have the most options. Make sure the campground is open and has water for the dates you've chosen. See if it's going to be busy. If it is, you can increase your odds of scoring the perfect site by being available midweek. If reservations are not available at your chosen campground, call or e-mail that district's ranger headquarters to see if the ranger recommends other campgrounds. All national forest campgrounds must be reserved at least four days in advance; for state parks the general last-minute rule is two days. Remember, if you arrive and don't like the reserved site, the campground host will move you if another site is available.

Next, get your equipment together. Everybody knows what basics to bring tent camping: a tent (of course), sleeping bags, a cooler, a stove, pots, utensils, a water jug, matches, a can opener, and so forth. But it's those little things that you suddenly wish you had that make for a really happy camper. The number one objective is a good night's sleep.

- **BRING EARPLUGS.** The first night or two out camping, the unfamiliar flap of the tent drives you crazy if you don't have earplugs. Also, a snoring mate sleeping a foot away from you is nighttime hell on earth. In addition, earplugs block out all that night nature stuff that interferes with a righteous camper's z's.

- **DON'T FORGET TO PACK YOUR OWN PILLOW.** A good pillow gets your shoulders off the deck and lets your hips and behind take the weight. Use your clothes bag as an additional pillow, and consider inflatable pillows sold at camping stores.

- **BRING A THIN FOAM MATTRESS OR BUY THOSE SELF-INFLATING PADS.** Buy some rubber shelf liners to keep your pad from slipping on the tent floor and keep your sleeping bag on top of it. Air mattresses are OK but susceptible to puncture. Don't expect a double air mattress to sleep two—every time your mate moves, you'll get tossed around.

- **GET A SLEEPING BAG THAT IS GOOD AND WARM.** Nothing is worse than being cold at night, and no sleeping bag is too warm. Just bring a sheet so you can sleep under it at first then crawl into the bag when it gets nippy.

- **PACK THE APPROPRIATE CLOTHING.** Check the weather: if it's going to be cold, remember to bring socks and sweatpants to sleep in. A sweatshirt with a hood is invaluable, since you lose a lot of heat through your head. Always pack a beanie.

- **BRING A WATER BOTTLE FROM WHICH TO DRINK AT NIGHT.** Consequently, a "pee jar" (a pee pot for ladies) just outside the tent is a great idea. You can stumble outside, use it, and empty it in the toilet in the morning.

- **BRING SOMETHING FOR OUTSIDE THE TENT TO CLEAN YOUR FEET ON.** Nothing disturbs your z's like grit inside the tent. In the woods, a square of Astroturf works fine. At the seashore or in the desert, a tray full of water in which to dip your feet works best. Bring a small brush for sweeping up whatever grit leaks in.

- **REMEMBER FLASHLIGHTS**. Mini flashlights work OK, and if you take off the lens, you can hang them from a tent loop and actually read. Be careful: The little bulb can get hot and will burn fabric or fingers. What works even better is a headlamp that straps to your head with an adjustable elastic band; you can buy them at any outdoor store. Everywhere you look, there's light. They're great for finding stuff, cleaning up in the dark after dinner, and reading.

- **PACK DUCT TAPE.** "If you can't fix it, duct-tape it" is a camping maxim.

- **BRING A SPONGE TO CLEAN OFF THE PICNIC TABLE**. A plastic table-cloth is nice, too (bring little pushpins to secure it so it won't blow away).

- **A PLASTIC BOWL OR AN INFLATABLE SINK** (around $11 at Walmart) is invaluable for washing dishes.

- **BRING A CUSHION**—picnic table benches get mighty hard.

- **BUY A CHEAP LAWN CHAIR,** and get the inexpensive umbrella that attaches to the back of the chair, so you can sit around the camp out of the sun.

- **YOU'LL WANT A FLY SWATTER** and mosquito repellent to wreak revenge on a lazy droning fly or fend off that irksome gnat in your ear.

- **BRING A LITTLE LEAF RAKE** to police your camp area.

- **REMEMBER BINOCULARS,** a bird book, and a wildflower book, so you can put a name to what you see.

- **YOU CAN USE 2.5-GALLON PLASTIC WATER JUGS** sold in supermarkets and refill them. They travel best with their valves up to avoid leakage.

- **A SOLAR SHOWER BAG REALLY WORKS FOR TAKING A HOT SHOWER.** After a day in the sun sitting on a hot rock, the water will be deliciously hot. Or bring along unscented baby wipes for a quick sponge bath. They work.

Don't be afraid to ask fellow campers for help or for stuff you might have forgotten. All campers know what it's like to forget basic stuff and love to help fellow campers. There's always a mechanic on vacation camping at the next site over when your car won't start, or somebody with extra white gas for your stove. Think heartily toward your fellow campers. Wave and say hi. And be sure to return the favor if a neighbor has forgotten something.

The campfire is an important camp event. Stores around the campground sell bundles of wood, and often the campground host sells wood. Also, there may be windfalls around the campground from which you can take wood (ask the campground host). You need a good **camp saw** for that. An absolute essential is a can of **charcoal starter fluid**. This guarantees a fire even in a driving rain. Naturally, don't forget **chocolate, graham crackers, and marshmallows** for roasting.

Fix up your car before you go. Nothing can be a bigger bummer than a mechanical breakdown on your way out. Have a mechanic check your water hoses and the air pressure in your tires before you load up. Remember, your car will be loaded down with stuff, and this will put a strain on your tires and cooling system. Bring an **extra fan belt**. Nothing can shut down the car like a snapped fan belt that you have to special-order from Japan. Even if you don't know a fan belt from third base, bring one. Somebody will come along who knows how to install it. **Make sure your spare tire is correctly inflated.** Mishap #999 is when you put on your spare, let the car down, and find out the spare is flat.

If you fish, be sure to get a license and display it. Fishing without a license is a misdemeanor, punishable by a maximum fine of $1,000 and/or six months in jail. On your way into the campground, stop at a local store and find out what the folks are using for bait. Buy it. This will save you a lot of experimentation and probably provide you with a good meal.

Remember the bears. Never leave your cooler out. Put it in the trunk, or disguise it with a blanket if you have a hatchback or a van. Don't eat in your tent. Put all cosmetics, soap, and other scented products in the car, and disguise them too; a bear will rip off a car door to get to a tube of lip balm. Bring a small bottle of bleach to wipe down the picnic table at night. Bears don't like bleach (but don't put too much faith in this!). If a bear raids your camp looking for food, beat on pots and pans and shoo it away like you would a naughty dog. And don't worry—even the boldest of bears won't dream of going into a tent unless it smells food inside.

Don't forget about mosquitoes. Where you have rain, trees, and rivers, there are mosquitoes, and they're hungry. Bring a couple of different kinds of repellent, as there are 3,000 kinds of mosquitoes. Repellent that some mosquitoes detest, others find very attractive. I like 3M's Ultrathon repellent—this is serious stuff. Sometimes, Avon's Skin-So-Soft works wonders; other times, it draws mosquitoes from miles away. A great idea if you are going to camp for a couple of days is a screen house. You can set it up over the picnic table or in a sunny spot and lounge in there while less-prepared neighbors are under siege. Coleman sells a lighter-duty one for just over $100, and Eureka sells a sturdier, larger one for, of course, many more bucks.

Come prepared for swimming. Bring old tennis shoes or buy water booties for wading in streams and lakes. Goggles are cool to check out what the trout are doing. Bring any rubber flotation device you can afford and carry in your vehicle that will get your highly vulnerable body on the gorgeous blue mountain lakes but out of the frigid water. Think air mattress with an air pump powered by the cigarette lighter of the car; they are lightweight and fun. Be careful not to set your device down on sharp shale or pine needles—and bring a repair kit.

Think about dispersed camping. With a fire permit, a shovel, and a bucket of water, you can camp just about anywhere in the national forests (consult the ranger district headquarters). The fire permit costs nothing, and there are miles and miles of fire roads and lumber roads you can explore to find the dispersed campground of your dreams.

FIRST AID KIT

A useful first aid kit may contain more items than you might think necessary. These are just the basics. Prepackaged kits in waterproof bags are available. As a preventive measure, always take along sunscreen and insect repellent. Even though quite a few items are listed here, they pack down into a small space:

- Adhesive bandages

- Antibiotic ointment (Neosporin or the generic equivalent)

- Antiseptic or disinfectant, such as Betadine or hydrogen peroxide

- Benadryl or the generic equivalent, diphenhydramine (in case of allergic reactions)

- Butterfly-closure bandages
- Elastic bandages or joint wraps
- Emergency poncho
- Epinephrine in a prefilled syringe (for severe allergic reactions to bee stings, etc.)
- Gauze (one roll and six 4-by-4-inch pads)
- Ibuprofen or acetaminophen
- Insect repellent
- LED flashlight or headlamp
- Matches or pocket lighter
- Mirror for signaling passing aircraft
- Moleskin/Spenco 2nd Skin
- Pocketknife or multipurpose tool
- Sunscreen/lip balm
- Waterproof first aid tape
- Whistle (it's more effective in signaling rescuers than your voice)

ANIMAL AND PLANT HAZARDS

SNAKES Northern California has a variety of snakes—including gopher snakes, king snakes, and racers—most of which are benign. Rattlesnakes are the exception, and they dwell in every area of the state: mountains, foothills, valleys, and deserts. The most common species found in the north of the state are the Northern Pacific rattlesnake and the Western diamondback. The whole of California has the sidewinder, the speckled rattlesnake, the red diamond rattlesnake, the Southern Pacific rattlesnake, the Great Basin rattlesnake, and the Mojave rattlesnake, according to the California Department of Fish and Game.

When hiking, stick to well-used trails, and wear over-the-ankle boots and loose-fitting long pants. Rattlesnakes like to bask in the sun when it's cooler and rest in the shade when it's hot (including on rocks, near water, and beneath picnic tables). They won't bite unless surprised or threatened. Do not step or put your hands where you cannot see, and avoid wandering around in the dark. Step *on* logs and rocks, never over them, and be especially careful when climbing rocks or gathering firewood. Always avoid walking through dense brush or willow thickets. Hibernation season is November–February.

TICKS Ticks are often found in brush and tall grass waiting to hitch a ride on a warm-blooded passerby. They are most active between April and October. Among the local varieties of ticks, the Western black-legged tick is the primary carrier of Lyme disease. To reduce your chances of ticks getting under your skin, wear light-colored clothing so ticks can be spotted before they make it to the skin. Most important, be sure to visually check your hair, back of neck, armpits, and socks at the end of the hike. During your posthike shower, take a moment to do a more complete body check. For ticks that are already embedded, removal with tweezers is best. Use disinfectant solution on the wound.

POISON OAK   Poison oak is rampant in the shady canyons and riparian woodlands of Northern California. It grows in moist areas, favoring shade trees and water sources. Avoiding contact is the most effective way to prevent the painful, itchy rash associated with these plants. Identify the plant by its three-leaf structure, with two leaves on opposite sides of the stem and one extending from the center. If you do come in contact with one of these plants, refrain from scratching because bacteria under fingernails can cause infection. Wash and dry the rash thoroughly, and apply calamine lotion to help dry it out. Remember that oil-contaminated clothes, pets, or hiking gear can easily transfer to you or someone else, so wash not only any exposed parts of your body but also clothes, gear, and pets, if applicable.

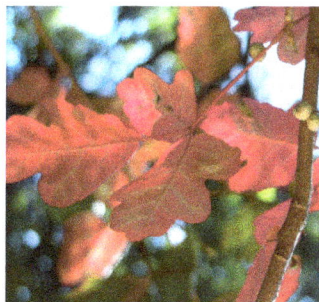
Poison oak foliage

photographed by Jane Huber

MOSQUITOES   Fortunately, in most of Northern California you're likely to have problems with mosquitoes only at dusk and dawn. The biggest exception to this rule is wildflower season. If you've happened to camp just before or during peak bloom, the skeeters may be unbearable. This is especially true in the Sierra Nevada and in Yosemite.

Though it's very rare, individuals can become infected with the West Nile virus by being bitten by an infected mosquito. Culex mosquitoes, the primary varieties that can transmit West Nile virus to humans, thrive in urban rather than natural areas. They lay their eggs in stagnant water and can breed in any standing water that remains for more than five days. Most people infected with West Nile virus have no symptoms of illness, but some may become ill, usually 3–15 days after being bitten.

Anytime you expect mosquitoes to be buzzing around, you may want to wear protective clothing, such as long sleeves, long pants, and socks. Loose-fitting, light-colored clothing is best. Spray clothing with insect repellent. Remember to follow the instructions on the repellent and to take extra care to protect children against these insects.

YELLOW JACKETS   Another pesky insect that seems to have exploded in many of Northern California's beautiful campgrounds is the yellow jacket, also commonly known as wasps or meat bees. Populations tend to peak in the late summer months, starting in August, and tenacious worker-bee activity doesn't stop until cold snaps in October.

If your campsite happens to be home to a nearby hive, there isn't much you can do to repel the wasps, but do take extra precautions: Be prepared to eat or prepare food inside a screened tent. Spend the $10 for a reusable yellow jacket trap. Lure the yellow jackets with scent-specific bait on a cotton ball inside the trap, to ensure you don't snag a beneficial honeybee, and hang the trap approximately 20 feet from your campsite. Unfortunately, people have died from yellow jacket attacks in recent years, so if anyone in your group is known to be sensitive to bee stings, carry an EpiPen for extra protection, and know how to use it properly.

SETTLING IN

When you come into a campground, be aware of a certain psychological barrier. This is a new place. You've driven all this way, and the campground doesn't look that hot. You feel disappointed. You feel like the new kid at school. The other campers look up from their game of gin rummy and hope you won't camp next to them as you drive around the campground loops and look helplessly at the open sites. Nothing looks good enough.

Park your car. Pull into the first available site that could possibly do. Then walk around the campground. You have half an hour to decide before you pick your site and pay. Once you get out and walk, you'll break through that "new kid at school" attitude and soon feel like you're a part of the place. It's odd: suddenly, you don't mind camping next to the gin rummy players. You realize that this is your campground as well as theirs. By the next morning, the whole place will feel like home, and the gin rummy players will seem like the best of neighbors. You won't understand why you didn't immediately recognize this campground as the best of all campgrounds.

When you plan a camping trip, try to stay in one campground for at least three days. Stay one day, and you end up spending most of your time packing and unpacking and getting familiar with the campground. Stay three days, and you'll relax and have fun.

Go tent camping. Live in paradise for a few days. Camping makes you want to sin like the damned, sleep like the righteous, and hike like the last of the great American walkers. It's a balm for the weary soul.

CAMPGROUND ETIQUETTE

Here are a few tips on how to create good vibes with fellow campers and wildlife.

- **MAKE SURE YOU CHECK IN, PAY YOUR FEE,** and mark your site as directed. Don't make the mistake of grabbing a seemingly empty site that looks more appealing than your site; it could be reserved. If you're unhappy with your site, check with the campground host for other options.

- **BE SENSITIVE TO THE GROUND BENEATH YOU.** Be sure to place all garbage in designated receptacles or pack it out if none is available. No one likes to see the trash someone else has left behind.

- **GIVE ANIMALS PLENTY OF SPACE.** It's common for animals to wander through campsites, where they may be accustomed to the presence of humans (and our food). An unannounced approach, a sudden movement, or a loud noise may startle them, and a surprised animal can be dangerous to you, to others, and to itself.

- **PLAN AHEAD.** Know your equipment, your ability, and the area where you are camping—and prepare accordingly. Be self-sufficient at all times; carry necessary supplies for changes in weather or other conditions. A well-executed trip is a satisfaction to you and to others.

- **BE COURTEOUS TO OTHER CAMPERS,** hikers, bikers, and anyone else you may encounter.

- **STRICTLY FOLLOW THE CAMPGROUND'S RULES** regarding the building of fires. Never burn trash. Trash smoke smells horrible, and trash debris in a fire pit or grill is unsightly.

HAPPY CAMPING

There is nothing worse than a bad camping trip, especially because it is so easy to have a great time. To assist with making your outing a happy one, here are some pointers:

- **RESERVE YOUR SITE IN ADVANCE,** especially if it's a weekend or a holiday, or if the campground is wildly popular. Many prime campgrounds require at least a six-month lead time on reservations. Check before you go.

- **PICK YOUR CAMPING BUDDIES WISELY.** A family trip is pretty straight-forward, but you may want to reconsider including grumpy Uncle Fred, who doesn't like bugs, sunshine, or marshmallows. After you know who's going, make sure that everyone is on the same page regarding expectations of difficulty (amenities or the lack thereof, physical exertion, and so on), sleeping arrangements, and food requirements.

- **DON'T DUPLICATE EQUIPMENT,** such as cooking pots and lanterns, among campers in your party. Carry what you need to have a good time, but don't turn the trip into a cross-country moving experience.

- **DRESS FOR THE SEASON.** Educate yourself on the temperature highs and lows of the specific part of the state you plan to visit. It may be warm at night in the summer in your backyard, but up in the mountains it can be quite chilly.

- **PITCH YOUR TENT ON A LEVEL SURFACE,** preferably one covered with leaves, pine straw, or grass. Use a tarp or specially designed footprint to thwart ground moisture and to protect the tent floor. Do a little site main-tenance, such as picking up the small rocks and sticks that can damage your tent floor and make sleep uncomfortable. If you have a separate tent rainfly but don't think you'll need it, keep it rolled up at the base of the tent in case it starts raining at midnight.

- **CONSIDER TAKING A SLEEPING PAD IF THE GROUND MAKES YOU UNCOMFORTABLE.** Choose a pad that is full-length and thicker than you think you might need. This will not only keep your hips from aching on hard ground but will also help keep you warm. A wide range of thin, light, and inflatable pads are available at camping stores, and these are a much better choice than home air mattresses, which conduct heat away from the body and tend to deflate during the night.

- **IF YOU ARE NOT HIKING TO A PRIMITIVE CAMPSITE,** there is no real need to skimp on food due to weight. Plan tasty meals and bring everything you will need to prepare, cook, eat, and clean up.

- **IF YOU TEND TO USE THE BATHROOM** multiple times at night, you should plan ahead. Leaving a warm sleeping bag and stumbling around in the dark to find the restroom, whether it be a pit toilet, a fully plumbed comfort station, or just the woods, is not fun. Keep a flashlight and any other accoutrements you may need by the tent door and know exactly where to head in the dark.

- **STANDING DEAD TREES AND STORM-DAMAGED LIVING TREES** can pose a hazard to tent campers. These trees may have loose or broken limbs that could fall at any time. When choosing a campsite or even just a spot to rest during a hike, look up.

A WORD ABOUT BACKCOUNTRY CAMPING

Following these guidelines will increase your chances for a pleasant, safe, and low-impact interaction with nature.

- **ADHERE TO THE ADAGES** "Pack it in, pack it out" and "Take only pictures, leave only footprints." Practice Leave No Trace camping ethics (lnt.org/learn /seven-principles-overview) while in the backcountry.

- **IN NORTHERN CALIFORNIA OPEN FIRES ARE PERMITTED** except during dry times when the U.S. Forest Service may issue a fire ban. Backpacking stoves are strongly encouraged.

- **HANG FOOD AWAY FROM BEARS** and other animals to prevent them from becoming introduced to (and dependent on) human food. Wildlife learn to associate backpacks and backpackers with easy food sources, which interferes with their natural behavior.

- **BURY SOLID HUMAN WASTE** in a hole at least 3 inches deep and at least 200 feet away from trails and water sources. A trowel is basic backpacking equipment; more and more often, however, the practice of burying human waste is being banned. Using a portable latrine, which comes in various incarnations (basically a glorified plastic bag) and may be given out by park rangers, may seem unthinkable at first, but it's really no big deal. Just bring an extra-large ziplock bag for additional insurance against structural failures.

VENTURING AWAY FROM THE CAMPGROUND

If you go for a hike, bike ride, or other excursion into the wilderness, keep these precautions in mind:

- **ALWAYS CARRY FOOD AND WATER,** whether you are planning to go overnight or not. Food will give you energy, help keep you warm, and sustain you in an emergency until help arrives. Bring potable water, or treat water by boiling or filtering before drinking from a lake or stream.

- **STAY ON DESIGNATED TRAILS.** Most hikers get lost when they leave the trail. Even on the most clearly marked trails, there is usually a point where you have to stop and consider which direction to head. If you become disoriented, don't panic. As soon as you think you may be off-track, stop, assess your current direction, and then retrace your steps back to the point where you went awry. If you have absolutely no idea how to continue, return to the trailhead the way you came in. Should you become completely lost and have no idea of how to return to the trailhead, remaining in place along the trail and waiting for help is most often the best option for adults and always the best option for children.

- **BE ESPECIALLY CAREFUL WHEN CROSSING STREAMS.** Whether you are fording the stream or crossing on a log, make every step count. If you have any doubt about maintaining your balance on a log, go ahead and ford the stream instead. When fording a stream, use a trekking pole or stout stick for balance and face upstream as you cross. If a stream seems too deep to ford, turn back. Whatever is on the other side is not worth risking your life.

- **BE CAREFUL AT OVERLOOKS.** Though these areas may provide spectacular views, they are potentially hazardous. Stay back from the edge of outcrops, and be absolutely sure of your footing: a misstep can mean a nasty and possibly fatal fall.

- **KNOW THE SYMPTOMS OF HYPOTHERMIA.** Shivering and forgetfulness are the two most common indicators of this insidious killer. Hypothermia can occur at any elevation, even in the summer. Wearing cotton clothing puts you especially at risk because cotton, when wet, wicks heat away from the body. To prevent hypothermia, dress in layers using synthetic clothing for insulation, use a cap and gloves to reduce heat loss, and protect yourself with waterproof, breathable outerwear. If symptoms arise, get the victim to shelter, a fire, hot liquids, and dry clothes or a dry sleeping bag.

- **TAKE ALONG YOUR BRAIN.** A cool, calculating mind is the single most important piece of equipment you'll ever need on the trail. Think before you act. Watch your step. Plan ahead. Avoiding accidents before they happen is the best recipe for a rewarding and relaxing hike.

THE COAST

Hike among the giants of northern California's lush forests in Jedediah Smith Redwoods State Park (*see page 48*).

Big Basin Redwoods State Park Campgrounds

Beauty ★★★★★ / Privacy ★★★★ / Spaciousness ★★★★ / Quiet ★★★ / Security ★★★★★ / Cleanliness ★★★★

Good tent camping, tent cabins, great hiking, marbled murrelets, and near Santa Cruz

This park is the granddaddy of all the incredible California state parks. Big Basin has wonderful camping, as well as tent cabins with interior wood stoves. Lovely Wastahi Campground consists of all walk-in tent campsites, with the farthest campsite 200 feet from the parking areas. Huckleberry is all walk-in as well, with the farthest site 50 feet from the parking areas. With Blooms Campground and Sempervirens Campground, Big Basin has another 102 developed campsites for RVs, but the park doesn't feel at all crowded. The huge redwoods give Big Basin a certain eerie calm.

On May 15, 1900, Andrew P. Hill camped at the base of Slippery Rock with 50 other conservationists. Together they formed the Sempervirens Club. Named for the *Sequoia sempervirens,* or redwood, the club was able to fend off the lumbermen and promote the creation of California's first state park from a deed of 3,800 acres of primeval forest. Now Big Basin has 18,000 ocean-facing acres of Santa Cruz Mountain full of redwoods, Douglas-fir, knobcone pine, oak, marsh, and chaparral, thanks to the Save the Redwoods League and the Sempervirens Fund.

Big Basin boasts 80 miles of roads and trails to explore the varied vegetation and watch for wildlife.

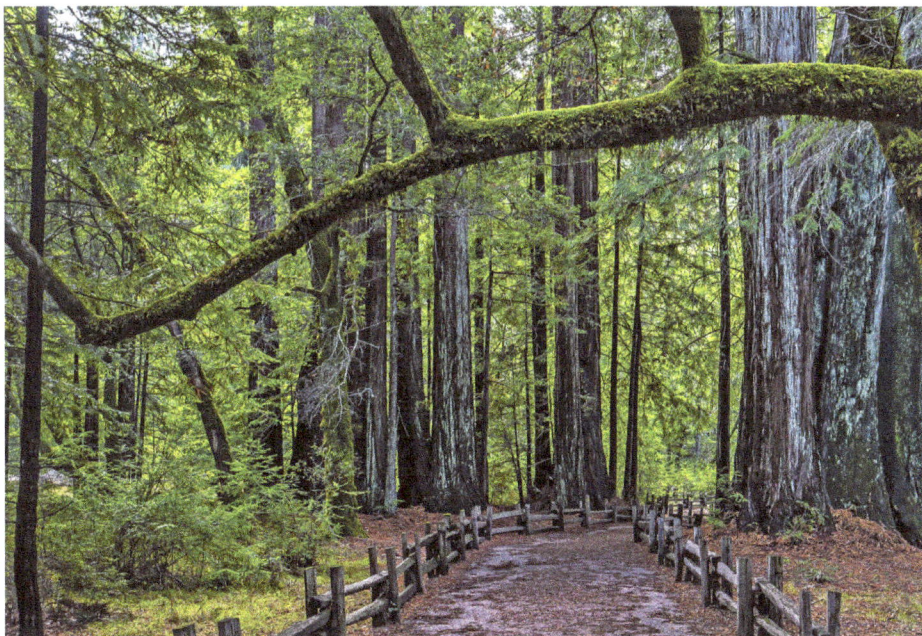

KEY INFORMATION

LOCATION: 21600 Big Basin Way, Boulder Creek, CA 95006

OPERATED BY: Big Basin Redwoods State Park

CONTACT: 831-338-8860; www.parks.ca.gov

OPEN: Year-round; some closed in winter

SITES: 142 total: 67 tent sites, 36 walk-in sites, 35 RV sites, 8 wheelchair-accessible sites, 35 tent cabins

EACH SITE HAS: Picnic table, fireplace

ASSIGNMENT: Online or by phone

REGISTRATION: By entrance; reserve campsites at 800-444-7275 or reservecalifornia .com; reserve tent cabins at 831-338-4745 or bigbasintentcabins.com

AMENITIES: Water, toilets, showers, firewood for sale

PARKING: At individual site

FEE: $35, $8 nonrefundable reservation fee, $10 extra vehicle

ELEVATION: 1,000'

RESTRICTIONS:

PETS: Dogs on leash only, in campground

FIRES: In fireplace

ALCOHOL: No restrictions

VEHICLES: RVs up to 27 feet, trailers up to 24 feet

OTHER: 14-day stay limit (7-day stay limit in summer), 30-day stay limit annually; 8 people/site; reservations recommended on holidays and summer weekends

To get to know Big Basin, you have to hike or mountain bike. Driving an automobile in these mountain areas is chiefly a white-knuckle blur of naked fear, brake lights, and squealing tires. Pull over, park the car, and put on your hiking boots.

First take the little Redwood Nature Trail loop to pay respects to an ancient redwood grove on the flat above Opal Creek. Look for azaleas blooming in early summer, and pick huckleberries in August. You'll see Big Basin's tallest tree, the 329-foot Mother of the Forest,

Big Basin Redwoods State Park Campgrounds

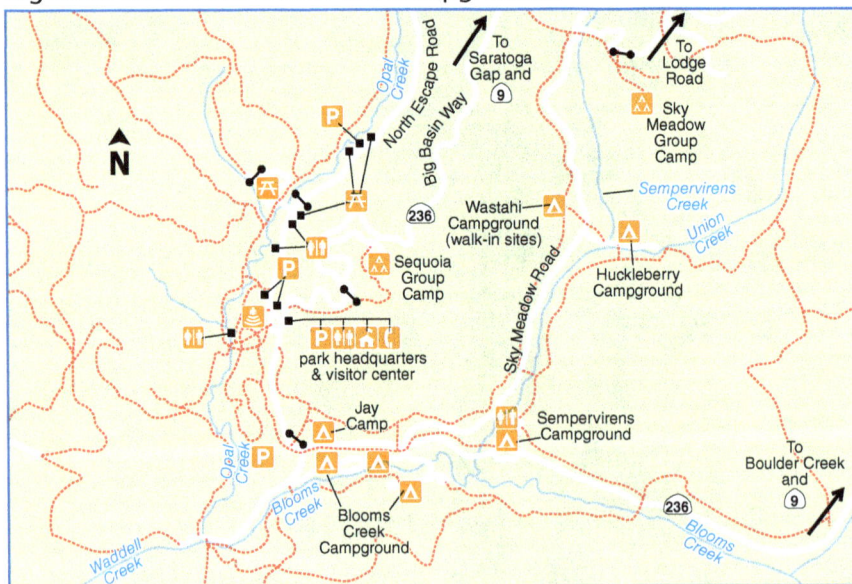

Blooms Creek Campground

Map labels: Sequoia Trail · To park headquarters · Sky Meadow Road · N · Campground Trail · 236 · To Boulder Creek · To East Ridge Trail · To Pine Mountain Trail · Blooms Creek · Blooms Creek Trail

Campsite numbers: 103, 104, 105, 106, 107, 108, 109, 110, 111, 112, 113, 114, 115, 116, 117, 118, 119, 120, 121, 122, 123, 124, 125, 126, 127, 128, 129, 130, 131, 132, 133, 134, 135, 136, 137, 138, 139, 140, 141, 142, 143, 144, 145, 146, 147, 148, 149, 150, 151, 152, 153, 154, 155, 156

the big-girthed Father of the Forest, and the Chimney Tree. Mother's roots pull up to 500 gallons of water up from the ground each day, which are released as moisture into the air—no wonder the forest is dank and lush.

Another quick hike is up the Sequoia Trail to Sempervirens Falls. The trailhead is right by park headquarters, and the trail is signed for Sempervirens Falls on the way up and park headquarters on the way back. The forest floor is bedded with ferns, and in the spring you'll see trillium, wild ginger, and azaleas blooming. Sempervirens Falls cascades by fallen redwoods into a crystal-clear pool. Round-trip, the hike is about 4 miles, though you can cut a mile or two off if you pick up the trail from Wastahi or Huckleberry Campground.

The 12-mile hike for which everybody comes to Big Basin is down to Berry Creek Falls. You start at park headquarters and hike through the redwoods, up over the ridge, and down 4 miles to magnificent Berry Creek Falls, with a 70-foot drop to a clear pool and more cascades fringed with ferns.

To get back, hike on up the staircase past Cascade Falls, Silver Falls, and Golden Falls, and follow Sunset Trail back to park headquarters.

Big Basin is home to black-tailed deer, raccoons, skunks, and squirrels. Rangers put up notices about mountain lions, but nobody ever sees the big cats. Even the American Indians called them ghosts. Marbled murrelets are as rare as mountain lions. These robin-size seabirds hunt fish in the ocean. Nobody had ever seen them nest until, in 1974, somebody discovered a murrelet nest made of live moss up in a Big Basin redwood. In bird-watching circles, a murrelet sighting is a great coup. Marbled murrelets are endangered in California for many reasons, including the proliferation of predatory birds such as ravens and jays in areas of old-growth redwoods. Jays and ravens are drawn to easy sources of food, such as that left behind by careless park visitors. Big Basin Redwoods State Park, as well as every

Huckleberry Campground and Tent Cabins

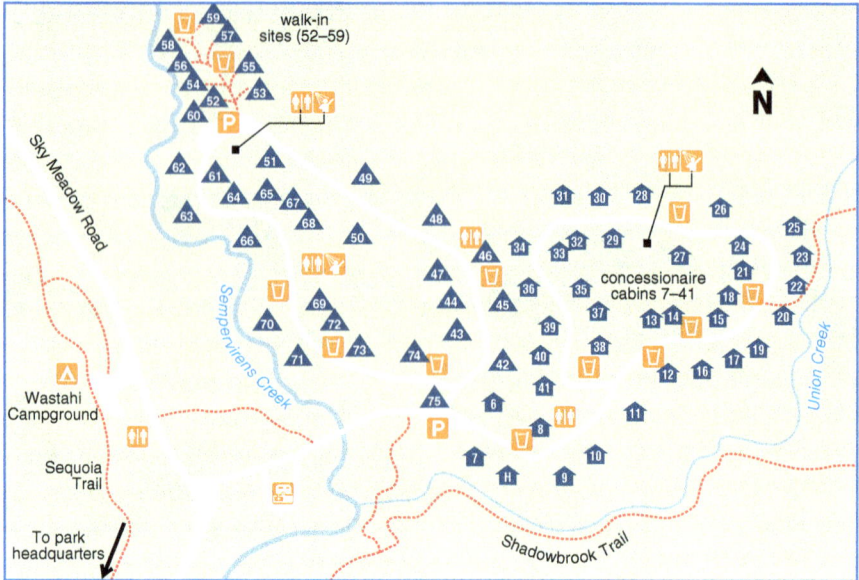

Sempervirens and Wastahi Campgrounds

California state park containing redwoods, has adopted a "crumb clean" policy for all visitors in hopes that the murrelet population will rebound as the jay and raven populations level off.

The nearest supplies are in Boulder Creek, but you want to go down to Santa Cruz and at least hike along the old 0.5-mile boardwalk. Kids will want to ride the undulating Undertow, the frenetic Fireball, or the thrilling Tsunami. Adults may prefer the Giant Dipper roller coaster (circa 1924) that comes from a more genteel era. Santa Cruz also has serious beaches, bookstores, a major university (even if the school mascot is the banana slug), brewpubs, and some good places to ea—like Aldo's at the west end of the yacht harbor.

Before you leave Big Basin, check out the 36 tent cabins on a loop road at Huckleberry Campground. Each has two full-size beds and a wood stove. Rent starts at $92–$145 per night, and additional camping packages and rental supplies are available. Next time you need a weekend off and don't want to mount a camping trip, these babies are the answer. Bring your own sleeping bags and pillows, and wood for the stove if the season is chilly.

GETTING THERE

From Santa Cruz, go north on CA 9 13.7 miles. Turn left on Big Basin Way and drive 7.7 miles to the Big Basin Redwoods State Park entrance.

GPS COORDINATES: N37° 10.338' W122° 13.320'

Big Basin State Park is the oldest park in all of California.

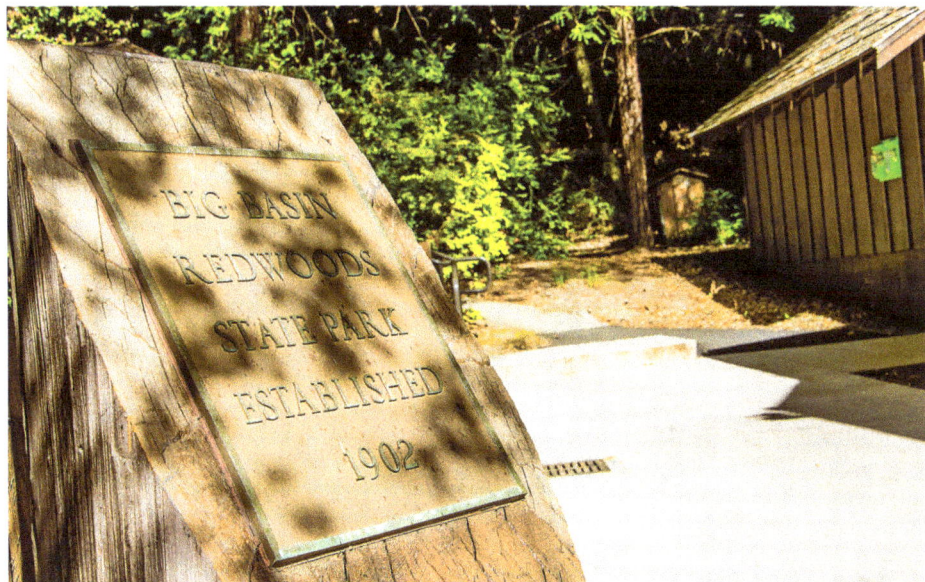

2

Butano State Park Campgrounds

Beauty ★★★★★ / Privacy ★★★ / Spaciousness ★★★★ / Quiet ★★★★★ / Security ★★★★★ /
Cleanliness ★★★★

Quiet as a church but with a carnival of outdoor activities around the campground

Drive along the windswept coast and turn inland on country roads baked golden in the sun. Turn up the canyon drained by Little Butano Creek and suddenly you are in a redwood rain forest—what an enchanted spot! Look for pygmy nuthatches, winter wrens, chickadees, banana slugs, and newts under the redwoods, Douglas-firs, tan oaks, maples, and ferns. This is prime camping, and most folks don't even know it's here. According to American Indian lore, *butano* means "a gathering place for friendly visits," and that's the vibe in Butano State Park.

The campground is up the canyon where the forest grows the thickest. Look for sites 22–39: these are the tent-only walk-in sites. At most, the walk is about 30 yards. The trees are so tall and the forest so still that camping here is like pitching a tent in a cathedral. The pitches are soft and spongy—although by fall there is a soft, red grit, so bring a drop cloth to clean your feet before entering your tent. The huge trees moderate the heat in the summer and the cold in the winter. Between the nearby rugged coast and these majestic trees, Butano State Park offers the best of two distinctly different worlds.

Hike up the Little Butano Creek Loop for a quick look at the park. The trail begins just below the campground. Cross the creek on footbridges, and look for trilliums, oxalises, and forget-me-nots. In the spring, look for baby newts. At a junction, stay below with the creek.

Sites 22–39 provide the most tucked-in feeling of the park, with sites beside the stately redwoods.

photographed by Luc Albarede

KEY INFORMATION

LOCATION: 1500 Cloverdale Road, Pescadero, CA 94060

OPERATED BY: Butano State Park

CONTACT: 650-879-2040; www.parks.ca.gov

OPEN: April 1–November 30

SITES: 35 total: 18 drive-in sites, 17 walk-in sites

EACH SITE HAS: Picnic table, fireplace

ASSIGNMENT: Reservations online or by phone; no walk-ups, site specific

REGISTRATION: By entrance; reserve at 800-444-7275 or reservecalifornia.com

AMENITIES: Water, pit or flush toilets

PARKING: At individual site

FEE: $35, $8 nonrefundable reservation fee

ELEVATION: 400'

RESTRICTIONS:

PETS: Dogs on leash only, in campground and on paved park roads

FIRES: In fireplace

ALCOHOL: No restrictions

VEHICLES: RVs and trailers up to 24 feet

OTHER: Reservations required on holidays, recommended on summer weekends

---

The paths soon come together and climb through the maples. About a mile out, either cross the creek and return to the campground via an access road or retrace your route.

A slightly longer walk is the Jackson Flats–Six Bridges Hike. Pick up this hike down below the picnic area by the entrance booth. Head up a ridge through Douglas-fir, madrone, and poison oak (don't touch). After a rain, look for chanterelle mushrooms (don't pick). After 1.5 miles, look for a cattail marsh on your left before entering old-growth redwoods at 2 miles. This is a good place to turn around. On the way back, one option is to take the Mill Ox Trail on the left and head back to the park road—go left uphill to the campground.

To visit the beach, go left on Cloverdale Road and down Gazos Creek Road to CA 1. Go across the highway and into the Gazos Creek access parking lot. There is a pretty little beach below Gazos, Whitehouse, and Cascade Canyons. Alternately, you can continue south exactly 1 mile. Park and walk over the dunes to the ocean. This is a great beach, with a protected cove at the south end and tidepools at the north end. A local showed me this beach and swore me to secrecy. Ha!

A little farther south find Año Nuevo State Park. This is truly an incredible experience. Northern elephant seals use Año Nuevo as a rookery. Spot the island and its abandoned buildings. This used to be a lighthouse facility, and folks who lived there often chased 2,000-pound elephant seals out of the kitchen garden and sometimes found them sliding down the halls of the house.

During breeding season, between December and March, male elephant seals as big as VW Beetles fight mano a mano for the ladies' favor. To see this spectacle, you have to take a ranger-guided walk, which requires advance reservations—as early as October. Phone 800-444-4445 for a spot. April–November, obtain a free permit, take a 3-mile self-guided tour through the reserve, and witness hundreds of seals and sea lions resting or molting on the beaches. The tour takes most groups around 2–3 hours. The pond is great for bird-watching, as waves of different birds pass through. The beach area is pristine and protected (careful of the rips), and the visitor center has a fine exhibit in an old barn, once part of the Steele Brothers Dairy Farm.

The charming town of Pescadero is a good refueling stop—this is one of the few spots for gas near the park. Arcangeli Grocery, on Pescadero's main strip, makes incredible artichoke-studded bread and other baked delights and stocks a small variety of grocery staples, meat, and poultry. Duarte's Tavern is a coastal institution, serving breakfast, lunch, and dinner in the same location since 1894. The cream of artichoke soup is justly famous, but the cream of green chili is also delicious; some folks ask for a mixture of the two soups in one bowl. For just-off-the-boat seafood, take a scenic drive north to Pillar Point harbor in Princeton, 4 miles past Half Moon Bay. If you'd rather linger near Pescadero, buy picnic fixings and head to Bean Hollow State Beach, where you can watch the waves crash on the shoreline.

Butano State Park: Ben Ries Campground

GETTING THERE

From Half Moon Bay, drive 15 miles south on CA 1 to Pescadero Creek Road on the left. Go east on Pescadero Creek Road, past the town of Pescadero. Go right on Cloverdale Road and drive another 4.5 miles. The park entrance is on the left.

GPS COORDINATES: N37° 12.704' W122° 19.835'

3

Salt Point State Park Campgrounds

Beauty ★★★★★ / Privacy ★★★★ / Spaciousness ★★★★ / Quiet ★★★★ / Security ★★★★ / Cleanliness ★★★★★

Sometimes in a campground, as in life, it's the little things that make all the difference.

Salt Point's campgrounds are a dream: impeccably clean, intelligently constructed, and full of details that show how much staff care about the park. These campgrounds are packed with little bonuses—water spigots painted to look like mushrooms, information boards with snippets about the natural life in and around the park, and fantastically clean, well-maintained sites and restrooms.

Situated on the rugged and beautiful Sonoma County coast, the park features more than 6 miles of coastline and more than 20 miles of hiking trails that wander through forest and grassy bluffs. The coastline here is a popular destination for abalone harvesting and features a protected underwater reserve where you can dive (no collecting). Trails depart from the campgrounds and lead about a mile (or less) to the beach. The two most popular hiking trails are the out-and-back coastal path from Salt Point to Stump Beach, and the loop through the pygmy forest. This pygmy forest, like others found along the coast, features dwarfed vegetation, and although the plants may look like they are struggling to survive, many of these shrubs and trees are more than 100 years old.

If you want more hiking, it's a short drive from the campground to the Kruse Rhododendron State Natural Reserve, where the main attraction is the park's namesake shrubs. They put forth gorgeous pink flowers in April and May. A fire swept through the woods on the south side of Salt Point State Park in 1994, and for years the hillsides were charred and

Ocean views span for miles on the hike between Salt Point and Stump Beach all the way to majestic Sentinel Rock.

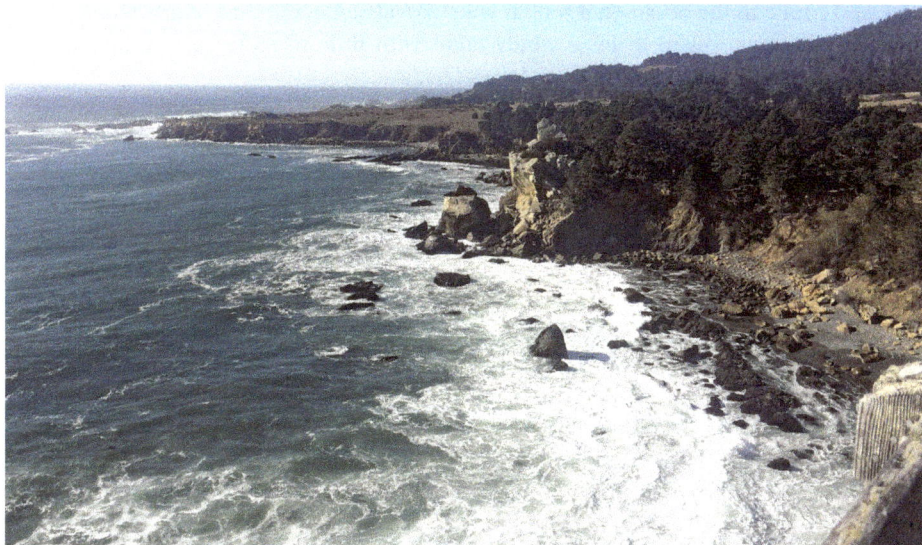

KEY INFORMATION

LOCATION: 25050 CA 1, Jenner, CA 95450

OPERATED BY: Salt Point State Park

CONTACT: 707-847-3221; www.parks.
ca.gov

OPEN: Woodside: March 15–November 30;
Gerstle Cove: year-round

SITES: Woodside: 79 sites for tents or RVs,
20 walk-in tent sites; Gerstle: 30 sites for
tents or RVs, 10 hiker/biker sites,
1 group site

EACH SITE HAS: Fire ring, picnic table,
food locker

ASSIGNMENT: Online or by phone; assigned
by ranger; walk-in sites are first come,
first served

REGISTRATION: At campground entrances;
reserve at 800-444-7275 or reservecalifornia
.com

AMENITIES: Drinking water, flush toilets, firewood, wheelchair-accessible sites

PARKING: At individual site

FEE: $35, $8 each additional vehicle, $8 non-
refundable reservation fee

ELEVATION: About 300'–400'

RESTRICTIONS:

PETS: On leash

FIRES: In fire rings

OTHER: Quiet hours (10 p.m.–6 a.m.) strictly
enforced; reservations recommended for
summer weekends and holidays

---

nearly denuded. More than 20 years later, young pines are reinvigorating hillsides, and the fire seems a distant memory; still, it's a good reminder to practice fire safety.

There are two campgrounds at Salt Point State Park, separated by a short stretch of CA 1: Gerstle Cove, on the west (ocean) side, and Woodside, on the east side. Gerstle is set on a bluff above the ocean, and the sites are generously spaced, but since there are just a few trees and hardly any other vegetation, privacy is slight. Our first reaction to Gerstle Cove was, "We love what they haven't done to the place." The sites blend into the beautiful natural setting of coastal grassland, with several downed trees that have been left where they fell. A few sites at the end of the loop are too close to CA 1 for our comfort, but sites 9–13 are prime, with the sound of the ocean to lull you to sleep. From the Gerstle Cove campground, it's just 0.2 mile to the ocean on a trail. If your arrival at Gerstle Cove is greeted by strong afternoon breezes, you're in for a windy night with little to buffer the gusts—consider Woodside instead; it is calmer.

The Woodside campground consists of two similarly sized loops: from the entrance station, lower Woodside is the first campground off the park road; upper Woodside is farther back and slightly uphill. After we settled into our lower Woodside campsite, we walked the campground loop a few times. Honestly, we would have been pleased with any of these sites—there's not a stinker in the bunch. All of Woodside's sites are well spaced, with plenty of vegetation screening views out of the campground. In upper Woodside, a few sites in the middle of the loop are open and grassy, but the rest of both campgrounds is dominated by bishop pine, Douglas-fir, cypress, madrone, and a few redwoods. Ferns, huckleberry, and salal make up the understory. In spring, look for irises, golden violets, and Labrador tea in bloom. In addition to ravens and Steller's jays (who will steal food left out in the blink of an eye), birds are plentiful, and we enjoyed waking up to the sounds of birdsong. "Go light" solitude seekers take note: In addition to the park's car-camping sites, there are 20 hike-in sites that are the quietest of all. These sites are 0.3 mile down a fire road or trail, and most are well shaded by dense redwood forest.

Salt Point State Park Campgrounds

Gerstle Cove Campground

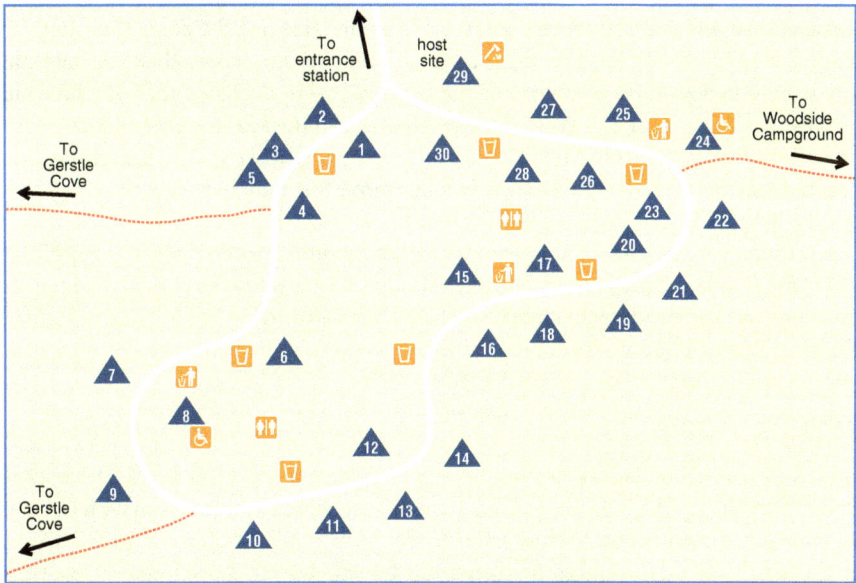

Woodside Campground: Lower and Upper Loops

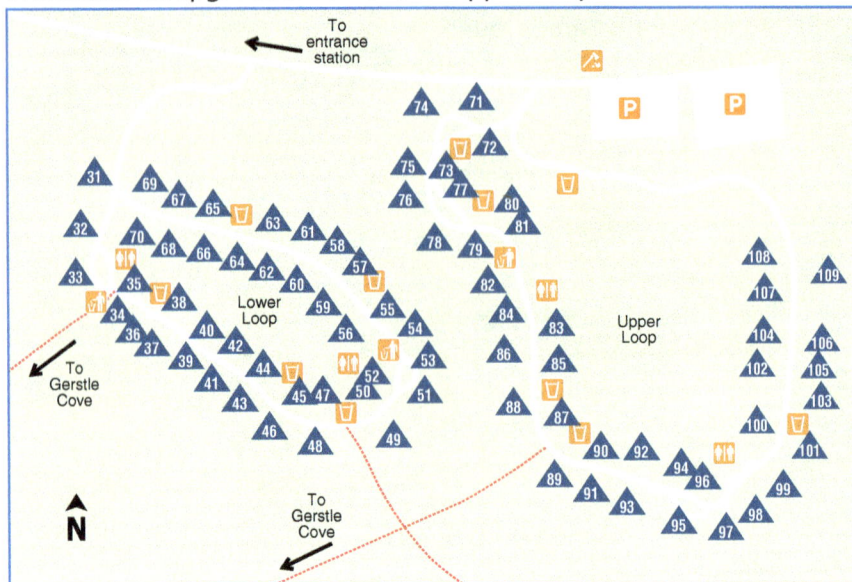

The weather along the coast is variable, but the general pattern is wet in winter, breezy in spring, alternately sunny and foggy in summer, and cool, calm, and clear in autumn. Reservations are recommended from mid-March to Halloween, but often the campgrounds are lightly used during weeknights. From our site, we watched the tall, thin bishop pines swaying in the wind and chipmunks scampering about. Heeding the posted warnings about raccoons, we stored our food securely, and although we never saw them, telltale muddy prints on the locked food container in the morning were evidence that our precautions were wise. If you camp at Salt Point in early winter, scan the seas for gray whales migrating south to breeding grounds in Mexico. Lucky watchers might see whales breeching, but you are more likely to see a few spouts as the whales move through. In spring the whales return to Alaska with their calves.

You can get gas and pick up supplies at the quaint general store at Stewarts Point (8 miles north of the park) or from a few small stores along CA 1 between the park and Jenner. These stores stock ice, firewood, snacks, and beverages, but there are no full-service supermarkets in the area. Bring your own fresh bread, meat, or vegetables from home.

GETTING THERE

From US 101 north of Santa Rosa in Sonoma County, exit on River Road. Drive 27 miles west on River Road, which becomes CA 116 in Guerneville, to the junction with CA 1. Turn right and drive north about 20 slow miles to the park. You'll reach the turn for Woodside Campground first, on the right; the turnoff for Gerstle Cove Campground is just 0.2 mile farther north, on the left.

GPS COORDINATES: **WOODSIDE:** N38° 34.148' W123° 19.257'
GERSTLE COVE: N38°34.227' W123°19.538'

4

Van Damme State Park Campgrounds

Beauty ★★★★★ / Privacy ★ / Spaciousness ★★★★ / Quiet ★ / Security ★★★ / Cleanliness ★★★★★

Come for the ocean, the whales, the pygmy forest, and nearby Mendocino.

Van Damme State Park lies along the most beautiful stretch of coast in America, where it doesn't snow during the wintertime. There is a sandy beach where folks actually dare swim, as well as whales, abalone, antiques shops, a pygmy forest, fabulous restaurants, and tent pitches on moss so soft you'll sleep like a baby. This is a well-run, friendly park. There are rangers, docents, and a campground host. Open all year, Van Damme is a park for all seasons.

Charles Van Damme was a Flemish kid who busted a gut working in a sawmill in Little River after the Civil War. He went on to operate the Richmond–San Rafael ferry, but he left his heart in Little River. When he finally got some bucks together, he bought 40 acres there and later willed them to the State of California. That land became the core of Van Damme State Park—now 1,831 acres of beach and upland.

Well before that time, American Indians lived along here as far back as 10,000 years. Of course, in those days, the sea level was 250 feet lower than it is today, so the shore where they gathered food was about 2 miles west in the briny deep, and the grassy headlands where we hike today were then pine forest.

Around 1587, a Spaniard on a galleon named this coast Mendocino for his friend back home—Antonio de Mendosa. A couple hundred years later the Russians came for the

Watch for whales December–May along the stunning coastline across the road from Van Damme State Park Campground.

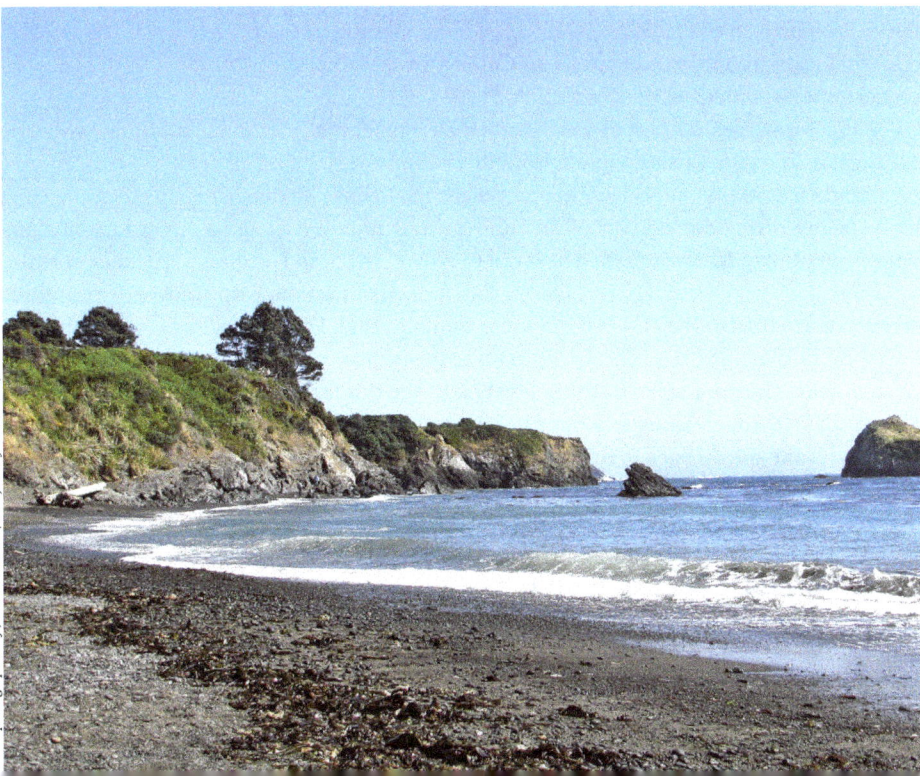

photographed by Jessica Fearnow (www.jessicafearnow.com)

KEY INFORMATION

LOCATION: 8001 CA 1, Little River, CA 95456

OPERATED BY: Van Damme State Park

CONTACT: 707-937-5804; www.parks.ca.gov

OPEN: Year-round

SITES: 68 sites for tents or RVs, 9 environmental (primitive) hike-in sites in Fern Canyon; 1 group site for up to 50 people

EACH SITE HAS: Picnic table, fireplace

ASSIGNMENT: First come, first served; reservations recommended

REGISTRATION: At entrance; reserve at 800-444-7275 or reservecalifornia.com

AMENITIES: Wi-Fi near visitor center, water, flush toilets, hot showers, firewood for sale

PARKING: At individual site

FEE: $45 peak season, $40 all other times, $25 for walk-in sites, $8 nonrefundable reservation fee

ELEVATION: 15'

RESTRICTIONS:

PETS: On leash only in campground, not allowed on trails

FIRES: In fireplace

ALCOHOL: No restrictions

VEHICLES: RVs up to 35 feet

OTHER: Reservations strongly recommended April–October; 2-week stay limit; up to 8 people/site

---

sea-otter pelts and were soon followed by the padres and the forty-niners, who were smitten by the beauty of the place and settled here after driving out the defenseless Pomo Indians. When J. Smeaton Chase, an eccentric English traveler, came through in 1911, he described the area as "such headlands, black and wooded, such purple seas, such vivid blaze of spray, such fiords and islets" and the town of Little River itself as "a pretty, straggling village of high gabled houses with quaint dormers and windows, and red roses clambering all about."

Little River is still pretty, and fun. The Little River Inn Golf & Tennis Club is open to the public, and you'll find food and spirits at the Little River Inn's restaurant and bar. Or go a few miles north to the fabled town of Mendocino, home to many restaurants, shops, and colorful locals. You may recognize it as Cabot Cove, Maine, the hometown of the fictional character Jessica Fletcher of *Murder, She Wrote.*

Watch for whales. It's best to look between December and May, in the morning, when the sea is calm. The gray whales migrate from the Bering Sea to Baja California, where they give birth to their 1,500-pound calves. Mama weighs in at about 30 tons. Look for them blowing water before diving down 100 feet for three or four minutes. To get a closer look at these behemoths, take a whale-watching boat out of Noyo Harbor in Fort Bragg (10 miles north).

There are a couple of decent hikes in the park. Head up the Fern Canyon Trail, which starts as a fire road at the east end of Lower Campground. Pass sword fern, redwood, hemlock, and fir along the canyon. By Little River grow alder, salmonberry, and thimbleberry. After 2 miles, the fire road ends (bicycles are allowed this far), and the trail goes deeper into Fern Canyon through Douglas-fir, redwood, and a plethora of ferns. The trail heads out of the canyon and circles back to the right, passing a redwood stump about 10 feet in diameter.

When you reach a junction with a dirt road, you can go left to the pygmy forest, where old-growth trees have 1-inch diameters and heights of 4 feet. Why? The soil is hard and mineralized, so the cypress and Bolander pine are stunted but produce an impressive crop of pinecones. In between these trees, look for tan oak and rhododendron, as well as blackberry and wax myrtle. Just beyond the pygmy forest is the Little River Airport Road, which heads back to Little River and CA 1. You can catch a ride back to camp or head back through the pygmy forest to the trail you hiked in on.

Back at campground central, take a stroll around the Bog Trail loop. This half-mile walk begins near the group camp where the forest meets the wetland. Watch out—the board-walks are slippery when wet.

The two campgrounds, Highland Meadow and Lower Campground, are only a few hundred yards apart. Between the two, I prefer Highland Meadow because it gets you up into the sun. Lower Campground tends to be dark and cool and gets the bicycle and foot traffic heading up Fern Canyon. Still, in the winter, it is the only campground open.

Be sure to reserve a campsite, especially for summer weekends; this coast is very popular. The beach is across busy CA 1, so be careful crossing—extra careful if you have children with you.

Van Damme State Park Campgrounds

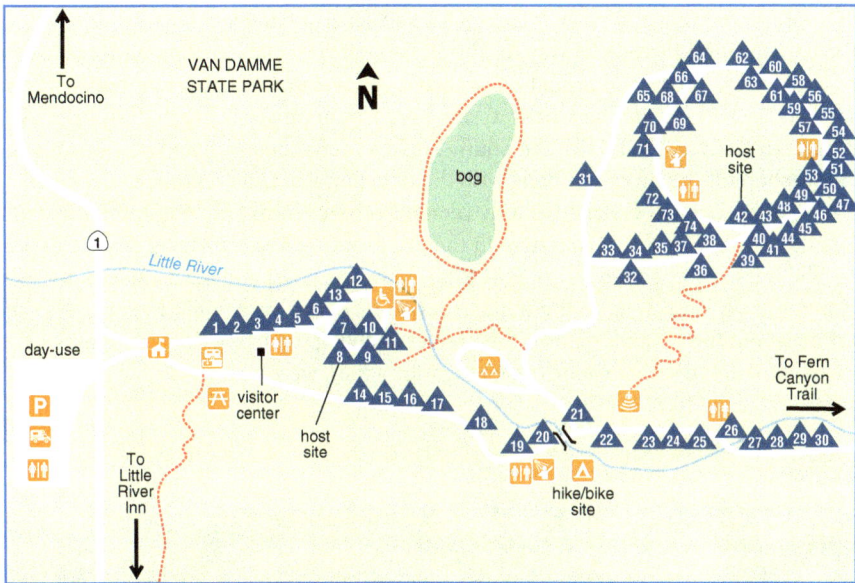

GETTING THERE

From Mendocino, drive 3 miles south on CA 1 to the Van Damme State Park entrance on the left.

GPS COORDINATES: N39° 16.448' W123° 47.438'

5

Russian Gulch State Park Campground

Beauty ★★★★★ / Privacy ★ / Spaciousness ★★ / Quiet ★★ / Security ★★★★ / Cleanliness ★★★★

Sits beside an azure gem of a cove next to the "jewel of the north coast," the town of Mendocino

Thank God for FDR and the New Deal, or we wouldn't have Russian Gulch State Park and the soaring arched concrete bridge that spans the gulch. What a pretty little campground! Take a left just after the bridge, and circle down a curved one-lane access road to the campground in the canyon and the beach across the stream under the bridge. The beach is all white sandbars, narrow blue water, soaring black cliffs spotted white, and green headlands. There is safe swimming and an easy launch for kayaks or inflatables.

The campground threads its way up the ferned canyon, with sites on either side of the access road. Cozy, mossy, and primal—that's what you feel tucked into a tent under the giant ferns, alders, redwoods, and hemlocks. Come here to sun on a safe beach. Fish for rockfish. Hike the Fern Canyon Trail. Hike the South Trail to Mendocino, where you can eat world-class food; shop till you drop; and hang with the rich, famous, and everyone in between.

Who named Russian Gulch? Nobody remembers, but local folks think the Russian fur hunters used to store bales of furs here in the otter- and seal-slaughtering days of the early 1800s. The Russians operated out of Fort Ross down the coast and used Eskimo hunters in bidarkas (sealskin kayaks) to do the stalking and killing. The local Pomo Indians, who knew something about the sea and the seals themselves (stalking them by painting themselves dark and pretending to be seals to get close enough for a kill), were amazed by the Eskimos' skill

The Frederick W. Panhorst Bridge on CA 1 spans Russian Gulch, a perfect place for swimming, launching a kayak, fishing, or simply watching the birds.

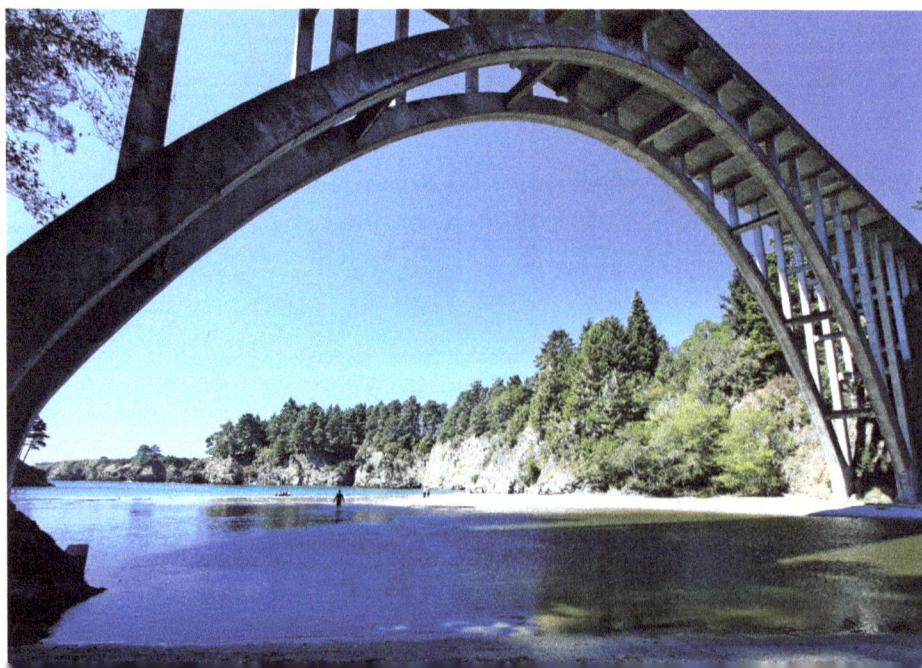

KEY INFORMATION

LOCATION: 12301 CA 1, Mendocino, CA 95460

OPERATED BY: Russian Gulch State Park

CONTACT: 707-937-5804; www.parks.ca.gov

OPEN: March–October (weather-dependent)

SITES: 25 total: 1 wheelchair-accessible site, 1 group site

EACH SITE HAS: Picnic table, fireplace, food locker

ASSIGNMENT: Reservations available late March–Labor Day

REGISTRATION: By entrance; reserve at 800-444-7275 or reservecalifornia.com

AMENITIES: Water, flush toilets, coin-operated showers, firewood for sale

PARKING: At individual site

FEE: $45 peak season, $40 all other times, $8 nonrefundable reservation fee, $10 extra vehicle

ELEVATION: 100'

RESTRICTIONS:

PETS: On leash only

FIRES: In fireplace

ALCOHOL: No restrictions

VEHICLES: RVs up to 24 feet and trailers up to 21 feet

OTHER: 8 people/site; reservations recommended in summer and on weekends; 15-day stay limit

---

in using their kayaks for the hunt. However, after the seals were mostly dead, the Russians packed up and headed home, leaving the Mendocino coast and the surviving Pomos easy pickings for a motley crew of forty-niners who followed the wreck of the *Frolic.*

The two-masted clipper ship *Frolic* sank off of Russian Gulch in 1850 with a hull full of Chinese silks and gewgaws. Henry Meigs sent his boys from San Francisco to salvage the wreck, but they found only happy Pomo women wearing skirts of Chinese silk and jewelry fashioned from oriental beads. Inevitably, Meigs heard about the huge redwoods in these parts and immediately sent a steam sawmill up to Mendocino to start ripping boards to build San Francisco, shore up gold mines in the Sierra Nevada, and make railroad ties for the Transcontinental Railway. The place boomed, with dozens of bars and hotels to entertain the hard-partying lumberjacks.

After that, Mendocino boomed, busted, and finally emerged around 1960 as the "jewel of the north coast"—a pretty little town full of arts, culture, great grub, scenic splendor, and a potpourri of Victorian Gothics, New England saltboxes, and false-front Western houses. I love Mendocino. People rag on it for being too cutesy, but I love it just the way it is—perfect for a couple of days of hanging out. The campground is an easy walk from town—just head up the South Trail where it leaves the beach road opposite the group camp. You come up over the bluffs then walk along CA 1 before taking the first right toward Mendocino.

Back at camp, hike the Fern Canyon Trail. This is a 6-mile round-trip trail that allows cyclists as far as the start of the Waterfall Loop. Head east through the campground. Look for nettles, salmonberry, and nightshade down by the creek, and alder, hazel, and laurel by the trail. After half a mile, you'll begin to see redwoods. At 1.5 miles there are some picnic tables. Beyond here, no bicycles are allowed. Hike up to the falls and admire their splendor. Then take the loop around to the right, back to the picnic tables, and retrace the trail back to the campground.

Another good walk is the Headland Trail. This 1-mile trail circles the park's north headland, showing off the incredible surf-carved rocks and cliffs. At the southwest end, look for a blowhole, fed by a sea cave, through which big waves blast up. Inland, look for the punch bowl where the roof of another cave collapsed. Plants hang over the rim, but the sea comes in through a small opening and washes the floor clean.

Good fun is canoeing the Big River. Call Catch a Canoe & Bicycles, Too! at 707-937-0273 to rent watercraft, which allow you to see seals, ducks, ospreys, and other wild critters. The Big River is an estuary, which means it's tidal, so you'll want to go upriver when the tide is coming in and downriver when the tide is going out. Go back to the jolly folks at Catch a Canoe and rent bicycles for a ride up Little Lake Road to Caspar Orchard Road and back.

While camping at Russian Gulch, shop at Harvest at Mendosa's.

Russian Gulch State Park Campground

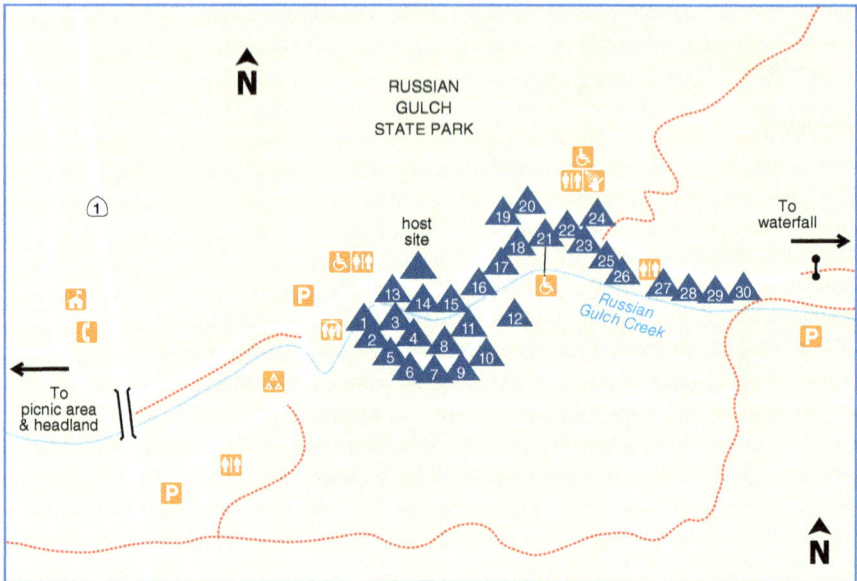

GETTING THERE

From Mendocino, go 2 miles north on CA 1 to the campground entrance on the left.

GPS COORDINATES: N39° 19.790' W123° 48.286'

6

MacKerricher State Park Campgrounds

Beauty ★★★★★ / Privacy ★★★★★ / Spaciousness ★★★★ / Quiet ★★★ / Security ★★★★★ / Cleanliness ★★★

MacKerricher State Park has everything but the promise of sunny weather.

What campground sits near 8 miles of beach, a beautiful headland, rolling dunes, lowland forest, a freshwater lake, and hundreds of snoozing harbor seals? MacKerricher State Park's campgrounds are cheek by jowl with all of the above.

The park offers hiking, cycling, surfing, canoeing, fishing, and horseback riding. Thank Canadian-born dairy farmer Duncan MacKerricher, who bought the land for $1.25 an acre back in 1868 and whose family later deeded it to the great state of California, specifying that access to the land be free in perpetuity.

The four campground loops—East Pinewood, West Pinewood, Cleone, and Surfwood—are pretty close together. East Pinewood is closer to the road. Cleone is a little closer to Cleone Pond. Surfwood is down by the beach but near the main beach traffic. I like West Pinewood best because it is off the highway and near the Haul Road Trail and an uncrowded beach. All the sites in all the loops are wonderfully separated and private. This is a first-class campground. There are 10 walk-in campsites (less than 50 yards away) in the Surfwood Loop for even more privacy.

More than just a pretty view, the coast at MacKerricher State Park is a great place for tidepooling, rock fishing, and seal watching.

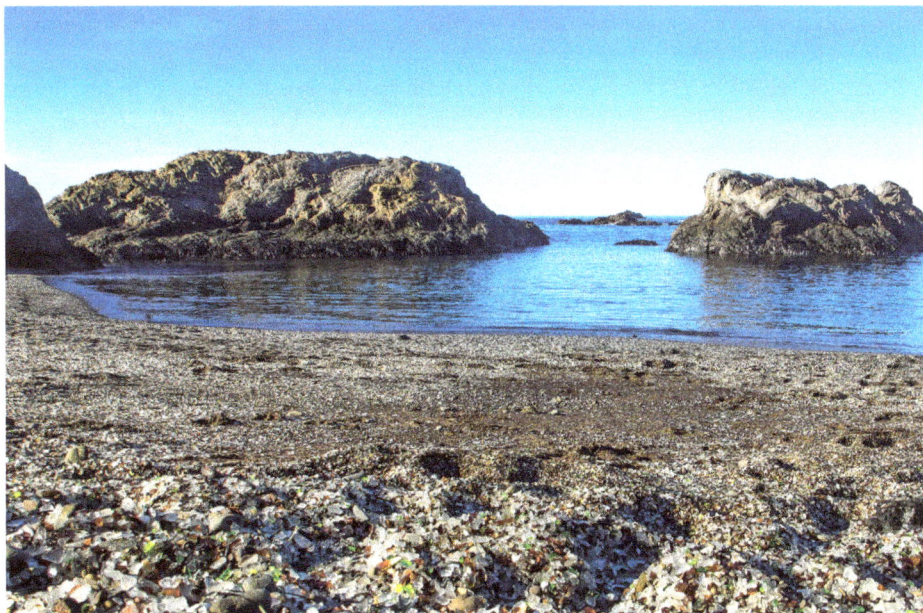

KEY INFORMATION

LOCATION: 24100 MacKerricher Park Road, Fort Bragg, CA 95437

OPERATED BY: MacKerricher State Park

CONTACT: 707-964-9112; www.parks.ca.gov

OPEN: Year-round

SITES: 120 sites for tents or RVs, 11 wheelchair-accessible sites, 10 walk-in sites (a 50-yard walk away), 2 group sites

EACH SITE HAS: Picnic table, fireplace, food locker

ASSIGNMENT: Reservations available March 1–Labor Day; otherwise first come, first served

REGISTRATION: By entrance; reserve at 800-444-7275 or reservecalifornia.com

AMENITIES: Water, flush toilets, hot showers, wood for sale, Wi-Fi access near visitor center

PARKING: At individual site

FEE: $45 peak season, $40 all other times, $8 nonrefundable reservation fee

ELEVATION: 50'

RESTRICTIONS:

PETS: On leash only

FIRES: In fireplace

ALCOHOL: No restrictions

VEHICLES: RVs and trailers up to 35 feet; 2 vehicles/site

OTHER: Reservations recommended in summer. Beach wheelchairs are available for use; call to reserve 7 days in advance: 707-937-5804.

Even though the campsites are protected by pines, brush, and ferns, come prepared for wind and rain. Weather on the Mendocino coast is unpredictable, though the scenery is often most beautiful when the weather is inclement. Sometimes, of course, the sun will shine for months.

Cleone Pond is perfect for launching a canoe or kayak, and is also good for trout when stocked and for some big, wary bass. The fishing here is relaxing, with the crash of the ocean waves only a sand dune away. There's a good mile's walk around the pond through marsh, cattails, and bishop pines.

Take the Seal Point Trail and hike a few hundred yards out on the walkway to Seal Rocks, where you should see tons of seals sleeping like sleek duffel bags on the rocks. Remember to bring binoculars to discern their cute little whiskered faces. Check out all the pretty spots on their creamy to dark-brown bodies. These critters spend most of their time copping z's, but they will all dive into the water at the sign of danger (an alarm bark). They can dive to 300 feet and stay submerged up to 28 minutes. Feeding time is when the tide comes in. Sometimes they head up the rivers with the tide to eat then haul out at low tide and snooze some more.

There is pretty good rock fishing north of Seal Rocks. Locals use squid for bait and tobacco-sack weights. The fishing stores sell little fabric tobacco sacks for next to nothing; you can fill them with sand or small rocks and tie onto your line. When the weight tangles up in the rocks, just give a pull and the tobacco sack weight breaks off, leaving you with your rockfish on the hook. Watch for rogue waves—the sudden big ones that come out of nowhere and threaten to suck you out to China.

It's fun, too, to go tide-pooling in the rocks at low tide. Or poke-poling! Here's what you do: Wear old sneakers and swimming shorts. Get a bamboo pole and attach a fishing hook on a 2-inch bit of wire to the end of the pole. Bait the hook with squid or mussels (rumors fly about the efficacy of abalone). Go around the tidepools in the shallow reef areas (best in minus tides) and stick the bait down under every rock and crevice. You'll get eels and rockfish and maybe small octopus. Serious poke-polers wear wet-suit bottoms so they can stay out longer. Bring a burlap sack for the booty.

Good bicycling awaits on the 10-mile Haul Road multiuse trail for hikers, cyclists, and equestrians. The first 2 miles are also ADA accessible. The route goes from the north side of Pudding Creek to the south, all the way north to the mouth of Ten Mile River. There's also decent cycling on the Fort Bragg Sherwood Road, which heads out in Fort Bragg as Oak Avenue. Great fun for everybody is the horseback riding. Ricochet Ridge Ranch in Cleone, just north of the MacKerricher State Park entrance, has guided rides on the beach or in the redwoods for very reasonable prices.

The campgrounds are right by Fort Bragg, which promotes itself as the town "where prosperity reigns and where it rains prosperity." Named for Braxton Bragg, a general in the Confederate Army, it was first a particularly brutal American Indian reservation. You'll find great seafood in Noyo Harbor, just south of town.

Go to the Mendocino Coast Botanical Gardens. The best blooms are in May, but something is always in season. Or ride the Skunk Train (707-964-6371; skunktrain.com) at the foot of Laurel Street. Antique railcars run 40 miles through the redwoods to Willits, crossing 30 bridges and going through two long tunnels.

MacKerricher State Park Campgrounds

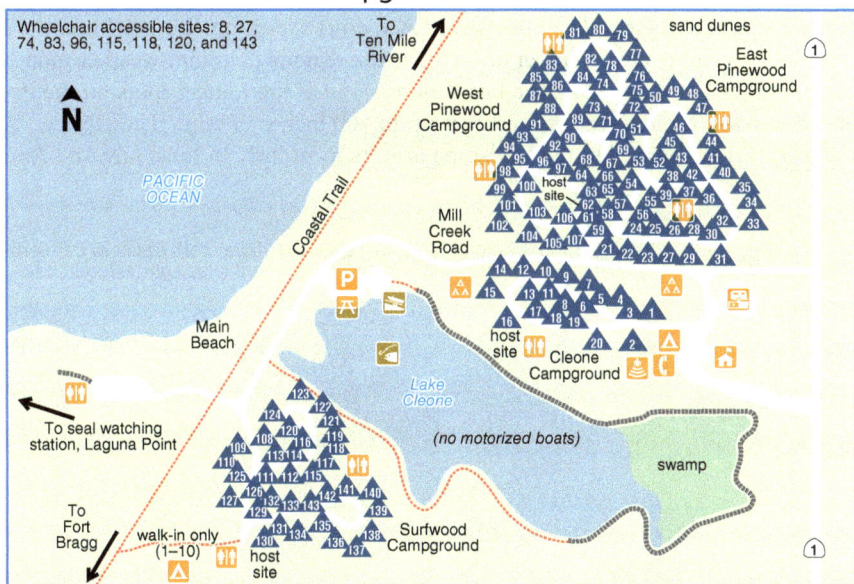

GETTING THERE

From Fort Bragg, go 4.7 miles north on CA 1 to the MacKerricher State Park entrance on the left.

GPS COORDINATES: N39° 29.333' W123° 47.469'

7

Nadelos and Wailaki Campgrounds

Beauty ★★★★★ / Privacy ★★★★★ / Spaciousness ★★★★★ / Quiet ★★★★ / Security ★★ /
Cleanliness ★★★★★

A good base camp for exploring the fabulous Lost Coast. Try to come in the fall.

These pretty little brother-and-sister campgrounds are right in the belly of the beast of the Lost Coast, where a fist of mountains rises straight out of the surf and black-sand beach. The terrain is so rugged that highway engineers had to route CA 1 many miles inland, leaving this huge hunk of land virtually untouched and begging to be explored. Nadelos or Wailaki campground makes a perfect base to do exactly that.

Almost on top of each other, Nadelos and Wailaki are virtually the same campground. Coming off Shelter Cove Road, Nadelos is first—the eight campsites are a short walk from the parking lot and are tucked into a hill across Little Bear Creek. Half a mile south is the entrance to Wailaki, which is engineered for trailers and RVs but is wonderful for tent camping as well. Last time I was there, both campgrounds were vacant, so we stayed at Wailaki, in one of the larger campsites. Both campgrounds have water and were recently reengineered, so the sites look clean and inviting, and the pit-style toilets are immaculate.

The valley is oriented north to south, so don't expect much sunlight at either Nadelos or Wailaki, except in the middle of the day. In fact, don't expect much sunlight on the Lost Coast unless you come in September or October, the region's premium-weather months.

From October through April, the Lost Coast is one of the wettest spots on the Pacific Coast. In wet years, the Lost Coast can get up to 200 inches of rain. That's 16 feet! April and May are often windy, and the landscape is at its most lush. In June, July, and August,

A short hike from Nadelos Campground, Chemise Mountain shows off flora that's distinctly different from that found elsewhere on the coast, as prevailing east-northeast winds keep coastal fog at bay.

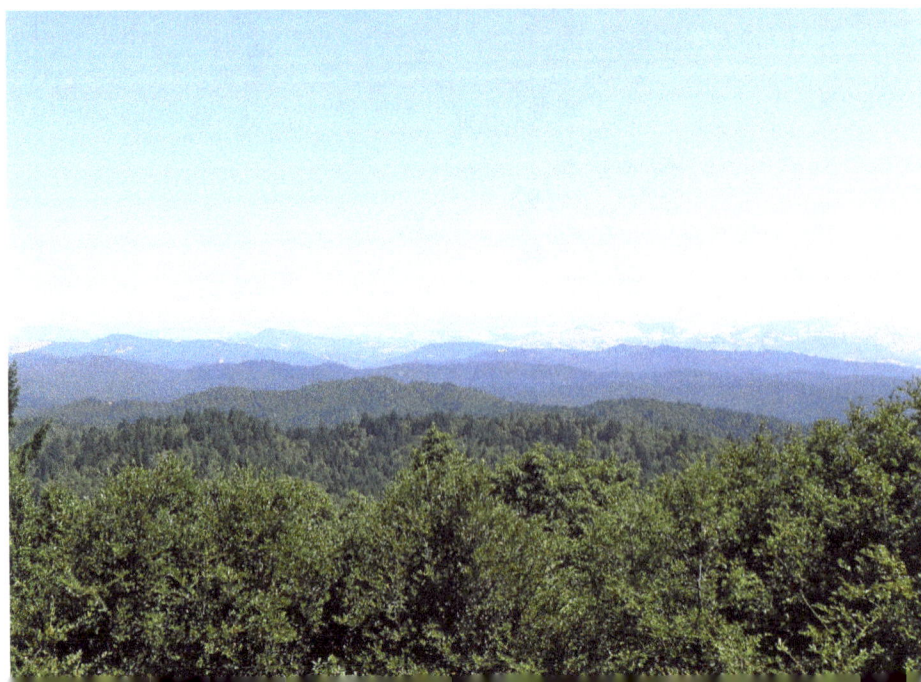

photographed by Rachel Sowards/Bureau of Land Management California/Public Domain

KEY INFORMATION

LOCATION: Chemise Mountain Road, 1.75 miles south of Shelter Cove Road, Whitethorn, CA 95589

OPERATED BY: King Range National Conservation Area

CONTACT: 707-986-5400; tinyurl.com /kingrangenca

OPEN: Year-round (depending on road and weather conditions)

SITES: Nadelos: 8 tent-only sites (entire camp can be reserved as group site—but not on Memorial Day, Labor Day, and July Fourth weekends); Wailaki: 13 sites for tents or RVs

EACH SITE HAS: Picnic table, fire ring

ASSIGNMENT: First come, first served; no reservations (except for reserving Nadelos as a group site)

REGISTRATION: At entrance

AMENITIES: Water, vault toilets; wheelchair-accessible sites at Nadelos and Wailaki

PARKING: At individual site

FEE: $8 site, $1 day use, $85 entire campground (20–60 people)

ELEVATION: 1,840'

RESTRICTIONS:

PETS: On leash only

FIRES: In fire ring

ALCOHOL: No restrictions

VEHICLES: RVs and trailers at Wailaki only (no hookups)

---

sunshine alternates with thick fog. Ah, but September and October are heaven. The hills are golden, and the sunsets explode across the sky.

Of course, tucked into the woods at Nadelos or Wailaki, don't expect to see the sunset. You have to drive down to the beach at Shelter Cove to see that. Shelter Cove used to be a giant sheep ranch but now has been developed into a real-estate nightmare. Retirees come in, build huge houses, go crazy from the isolation of the Lost Coast, and run screaming back to civilization. So there are lots of big houses going for very few dollars at Shelter Cove.

There are wonderful beaches as well. Black Sands Beach at the north end of town basically continues 24 miles north to the mouth of the Mattole River. This is a famous hike that folks usually take from north to south because of the prevailing winds. Hikers should bring water (or a water-purifying device), a tidal schedule to time certain beaches, and camping equipment. In town, find the short trail to Little Black Sands Beach, which is a favorite of the locals. And, of course, south of town past the Shelter Cove Marina and Campground is Dead Man's Beach—famous among beach people.

Nearby, be sure to stop at the Shelter Cove General Store, which has a great selection of beer and wine, and definitely don't miss the fish-and-chips at the Shelter Cove Campground Deli. The fish is incredible—caught fresh every morning. The chips are thick and light. The portions are enormous. I asked for a half portion, and the tiny woman at the counter laughed. "If I can eat a whole order, so can you!" she said, and she was right. I sat outside at the picnic tables with my fish and chips and beer, with the sun setting on the Pacific Ocean before me.

At both Nadelos and Wailaki Campgrounds, you'll spot signed trails that head west to both the Lost Coast Trail and the Hidden Valley Trail. The Hidden Valley Trail heads north 1.75 miles to the Chemise Mountain Road, where you can walk back south past the little cabins to the campgrounds. The trail south goes to Chemise Mountain (3 miles round-trip) and Whale Gulch (10 miles round-trip). Look for a herd of transplanted Roosevelt elk along the way.

Bring water. The nearest water on the Whale Gulch Trail is at the Needle Rock visitor center 6 miles away. It's not a bad idea to stash a car or arrange a pickup at the visitor center for the trip back. (To reach Needle Rock from the campgrounds, head south on Chemise Mountain Road to Four Corners, then go right on Briceland Road to Needle Rock.)

If you're in a thrill-seeking mood, bring a mountain bike to ride all or some of the Paradise Royale Trail System's 23 miles of swooping singletrack. Referred to as some of Northern California's best, you'll find varied levels of developed bike park features along with dramatic vistas and a true wilderness-mountain-biking feel. From Shelter Cove Road, turn north on King Peak Road. You'll find Tolkan Campground and trailhead access in 3.5 miles.

For a grueling but fun road trip, turn south on Usal Road at Four Corners and drive down to Usal Beach and CA 1. Phone the Sinkyone Wilderness State Park at 707-247-3318 to get a reading on the road conditions. Impassable in winter, this road hasn't changed much since Jack London and his wife, Charmian, came up in a wagon in 1911.

Nadelos and Wailaki Campgrounds

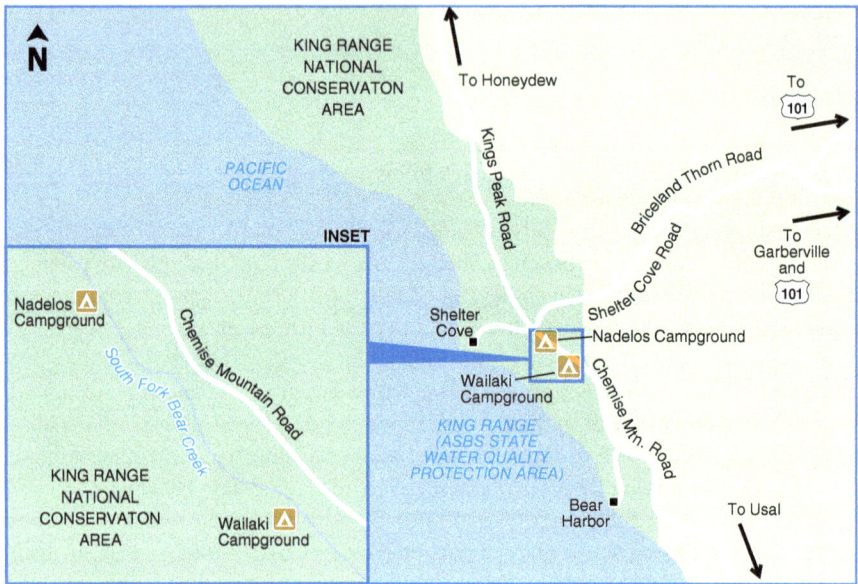

GETTING THERE

From Redway (northeast of Garberville on US 101), drive 12 miles west on Briceland Thorn Road; veer slightly right as the road becomes Shelter Cove Road, and continue about another 5 miles. Go 1.75 miles south on Chemise Mountain Road to Nadelos Campground, then another 0.5 mile south to Wailaki Campground.

GPS COORDINATES: **NADELOS:** N40° 1.151' W124° 0.199'
WAILAKI: N40° 1.070' W124° 0.081'

8

Patrick's Point State Park:
AGATE, PENN, AND ABALONE CAMPGROUNDS

Beauty ★★★★★ / Privacy ★★★★★ / Spaciousness ★★★★ / Quiet ★★★ / Security ★★★★★ /
Cleanliness ★★★★★

Patrick's Point Campground has everything—beauty, sea lions, an American Indian village, and hot clam chowder nearby.

Most beautiful of all California's state parks, Patrick's Point is full of enchanted Sitka-spruce groves and dizzying cliffs running down to ancient sea stacks, sea lions, and the foaming green Pacific. The three campground loops in the park, Agate, Penn, and Abalone, are under trees, the campsites nestled in bracken fern, sword fern, and salmonberry. The Sitkas, with their silver moss, crinkled bark, and golden cones, loom out of the mist. Each site is private, secluded, and special. On the beach, find agates and sometimes jade. Surf fish for perch and flounder. With the Yurok Indian village of Sumeg in the park, and Trinidad nearby with the marine lab and party fishing boats, there's lots to do with kids.

Take the Rim Trail to get a sense of the headlands. Accessible from various places, the trail goes 2 miles around the promontory, passing little trails to Palmer's Point, Abalone Point, Rocky Point, Patrick's Point, Wedding Rock, and Mussel Rocks. By the time you take all these spur trails, the trip is more like 4 miles. Wedding Rock is a good place to look for whales during the season.

Head to Palmer's Point and climb down to the tide-pool area. Look for sea lions and harbor seals. The sea lions are bigger than the seals, without spots, and their buff to brown hide looks black when it is wet. Sea lions are the fastest swimmers—up to 25 miles per hour when pressed. They can descend to 450 feet and stay submerged for 20 minutes.

Wedding Rock is a prominent outcrop along the coast at Patrick's Point State Park. It is an excellent place for spotting California gray whales November–April and also host weddings (707-677-3110).

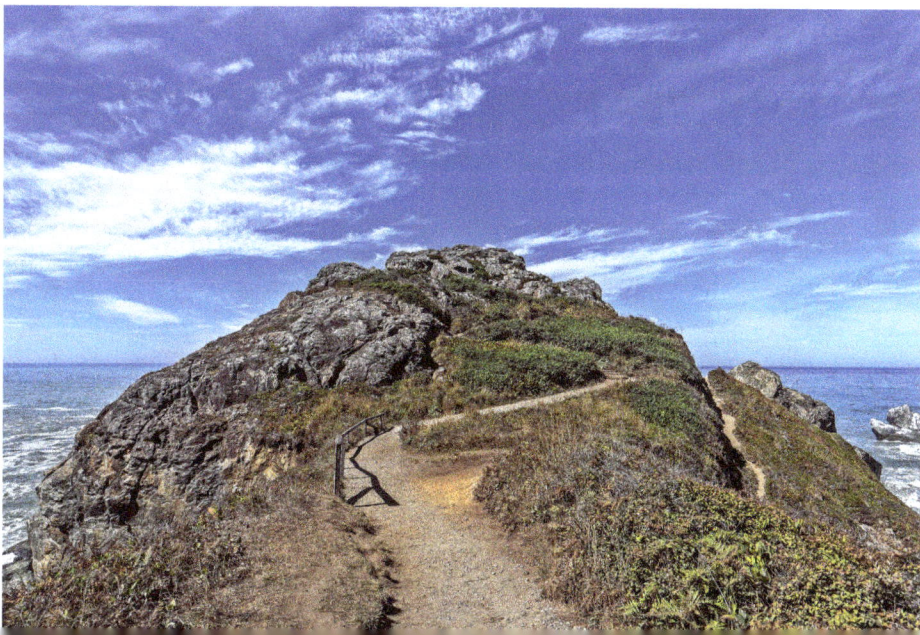

LOCATION: 4150 Patrick's Point Drive, Trinidad, CA 95570

OPERATED BY: Patrick's Point State Park

CONTACT: 707-677-3570; www.parks.ca.gov

OPEN: Year-round

SITES: 121 sites for tents or RVs, 2 group sites, environmental camp for hikers and cyclists; tent cabins also available

EACH SITE HAS: Picnic table, fireplace, food locker

ASSIGNMENT: Assigned by ranger

REGISTRATION: By entrance; reserve at 800-444-7275 or reservecalifornia.com

AMENITIES: Water, flush toilets, coin-operated showers, firewood for sale

PARKING: At individual site

FEE: $35, $8 extra vehicle, $8 nonrefundable reservation fee

ELEVATION: 100'

RESTRICTIONS:

PETS: On leash only in campground, not on the trails

FIRES: In fireplace

ALCOHOL: No restrictions

VEHICLES: RVs up to 31 feet

OTHER: First come, first served Labor Day–Memorial Day; reservations recommended during peak season

Hike down to Agate Beach, where the agate finding is easiest after a high tide. The best hunting, though, is after a winter storm. The agates found here are unpolished and look just like little white-and-bluish quartz stones. Take them home and put them in a bottle with oil so they always look wet and pretty. Keep hiking 2 miles and come to Humboldt Lagoons State Park. These lagoons are the sand-drowned mouths of streams. Spits of wave-borne sand form across their outlets to dam up the streams until the ocean cuts a floodgate through. Check out the dunes for beach pea, salt grass, verbena, and sea rocket. On

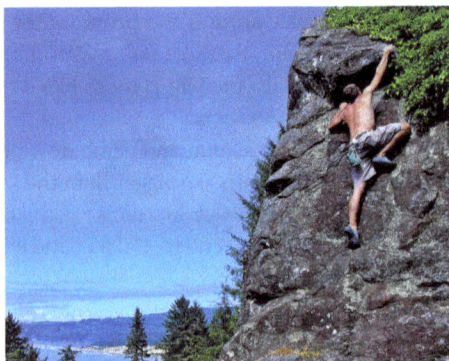

Patrick's Point State Park has more than a dozen classic climbing routes (mostly trad and top rope).

the shore is more Sitka spruce, red alder, and redwood. This was prime Yurok country.

The Yuroks moved between fishing and hunting camps. They trapped elk in deep pits covered with branches and dirt, and they speared sea lions by painting their own bodies dark and wriggling up close enough for the kill. They netted ducks and geese and gill-netted salmon. The women gathered acorns, leached them, and made bread. Dried eel was a specialty (a big hit with hungry European explorers). Abalone was an everyday staple, as well as edible seaweed. The Yuroks lived well.

At the foot of the lagoons is Big Lagoon County Park, with a boat ramp for canoers, kayakers, and windsurfers. Consider the tent camping here for another trip or if Patrick's Point is jammed up. You are at water ground zero just off the Big Lagoon. The tent pitches are grassy sand. There's good camping (no reservations) but not much of the cover privacy that Patrick's Point has in spades. I talked to the ranger there who said the fishing is pretty slim until the ocean cuts through the dunes. Then you get steelhead, sea-run cutthroat trout, sharks, flounder, and so on. To drive to Big Lagoon County Park from Patrick's Point, just go 1 mile north on US 101. Turn left at Big Lagoon Road and follow the signs.

Another good trip is to nearby Trinidad. Everyone likes the Humboldt State University Marine Lab and Aquarium (open weekdays year-round and weekends during the academic year). Sir Francis Drake once anchored at this old whaling town, which now offers peerless clam chowder and cod sandwiches at the Seascape Restaurant down on the Trinidad Wharf. The fish come off the fishing boats and directly through the kitchen door of Seascape.

Come here in July and go for salmon. There are charter and party boats available, and the fish are sometimes close enough for small boats. A word of warning though: This coast is notorious for fogging in, so watch your navigation or you'll end up in Hawaii.

No luck fishing? Stop at Katy's Smokehouse on Edwards Street across from the Trinidad Memorial Lighthouse to buy fish or crab to take back to camp. When the Dungeness come in November, Katy's is crab-lovers' heaven, and the smoked albacore is incomparable.

The Yuroks revered Patrick's Point and believed that the spirit of the porpoises lived here and that the seven sea stacks were the last earthly abode of the immortals. Patrick Beegan, an Irishman who came here in 1851, just liked the wild Indian potatoes (lily bulbs) that grew here; hence the name Patrick's Point.

Patrick's Point State Park Campgrounds

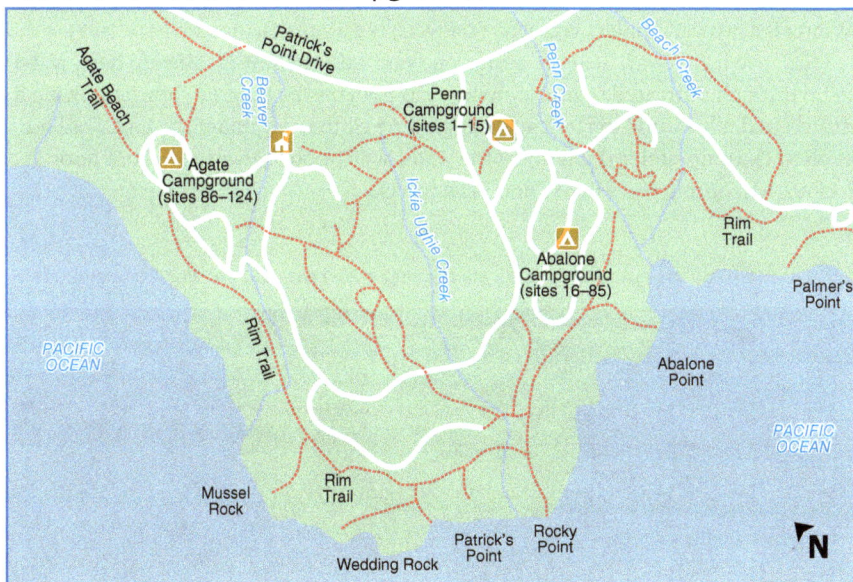

GETTING THERE

From Trinidad, go 6 miles north on US 101 to the Patrick's Point State Park entrance on the left.

GPS COORDINATES: N41° 8.167' W124° 9.605'

9

Elk Prairie Campground

Beauty ★★★★★ / Privacy ★★★★★ / Spaciousness ★★★ / Quiet ★★★ / Security ★★★★★ / Cleanliness ★★★★★

Redwoods, the beach, and the elk will amuse the kids on a summer family vacation.

This pretty campground is perfect for families. Just off US 101, it has all the amenities—flush toilets, hot showers, secluded campsites set off in redwoods and maples, and a meadow full of child-pleasing wapiti, otherwise known as elk. These huge animals, *Cervus elaphus* (or Roosevelt elk, in honor of Teddy, the president who helped protect them), are instant crowd-pleasers. Cars come to a screeching halt when they appear beside the road. Kids are fascinated by their huge antlers, and the baby elk would melt anyone's heart.

The trails are many and easy—and free of poison oak! A few miles away (by car or on foot) is Gold Bluffs Beach, the most beautiful, most secluded sandy beach in all of California. Orick, a few miles south, has all the redwood burls the world could ever desire, along with basic groceries and supplies.

The absolute best time to come is in September and October, when the sun shines. Summer is warmer, but expect some fog, and be prepared to dress for it. Spring has rainy spells but also wildflowers.

Winter is a bear, and unless you arrive between huge storms, prepare to be wet—although some folks love it this way. Seal the seams on your tent; the way it rains up here, water will come up through untreated seams to make a lap pool on the floor of your tent. Bring a garden trowel to ditch around the tent and a good drop cloth to lay under the tent. Fold the sides of the drop cloth up under the tent, so the water won't pool between the tent floor and the drop cloth. Also, bring good books and playing cards.

Tune into AM 1610 to find out where the elk are roaming in and around Elk Prairie Campground.

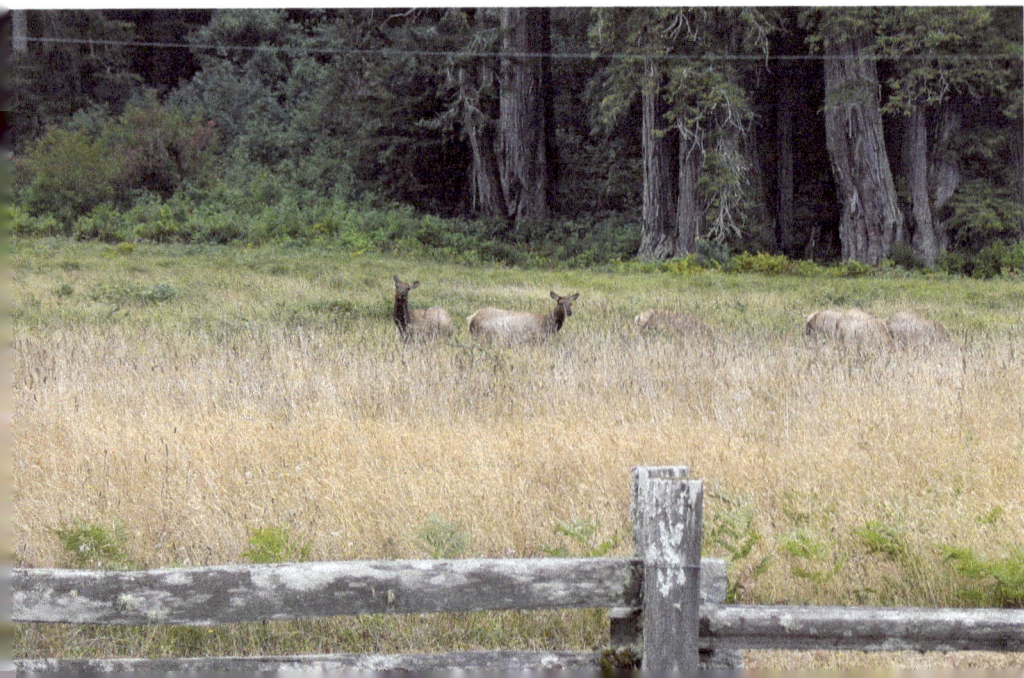

KEY INFORMATION

LOCATION: 127077 Newton B. Drury Scenic Parkway, Orick, CA 95555

OPERATED BY: Prairie Creek Redwoods State Park and National Park Service

CONTACT: Visitor center 707-488-2039; camping kiosk 707-488-2171; www.parks.ca.gov

OPEN: Year-round

SITES: 61 sites for tents or RVs, 4 wheelchair-accessible sites, 4 cabins (all wheelchair accessible; see 44 for more on cabins)

EACH SITE HAS: Picnic table, fire ring, food locker

ASSIGNMENT: Reservations recommended May–September; otherwise first come, first served

REGISTRATION: By entrance; reserve at 800-464-7275 or reservecalifornia.com

AMENITIES: Water, flush toilets, showers, firewood for sale

PARKING: At individual site

FEE: $35, $8 nonrefundable reservation fee

ELEVATION: 150'

RESTRICTIONS:

PETS: On leash only

FIRES: In fire ring

ALCOHOL: No restrictions

VEHICLES: RVs up to 27 feet, trailers up to 24 feet

The elk don't mind the wet. They're just glad not to be hunted to near extinction for their meat, hide, and upper canine teeth. At one time, these elk ranged over most of the continent—from the Berkshires in western Massachusetts to southern New Mexico. By 1912, the herd was down to about 15 elk. They made their last stand here in Prairie Creek Redwoods State Park.

Elk love elk. Very gregarious, these animals band together even at the risk of running out of pasture. Known for their huge, intimidating antlers, the bulls are paper tigers; the antlers seem to be mostly for show. When they fight, they strike with their front feet and use the antlers in a chopping, downward motion. Most important for the bull elk is his bugle—beginning low and rising a full octave to a sweet, mellow crescendo; dropping by degrees to the first note; and culminating with a few coughing grunts. The bulls here are big bark and little bite. Of course, humanoids should not approach elk or get in their way.

Listen to AM radio 1610 while in the park. This is elk local news and will tell you where the herd is. A good elk-spotting hike is around Elk Prairie. Bring binoculars. A little more than 2 miles long, the loop should take a little over an hour. Start near campsite 67 and follow the trail south through Sitka spruce and alder. Cross a little stream, then head into the open prairie. At a break in the fence, head across the prairie to the parkway, cross it, and pick up the trail on the other side. This trail will parallel the parkway. Look for signs of elk—tracks, bark rubbed off, tender shoots eaten, elk wallows—and the elk herd itself. Keep going until you reach a junction with the Rhododendron and Cathedral Trees Trails. Go left and circle back to the campground, going under the parkway by the kiosk and visitor center.

Another good hike is down to Fern Canyon and the beach via the James Irvine Trail. This is a day hike, about 8 miles round-trip, so take water and food. To pick up the James Irvine Trail, take the nature trail by the visitor center, cross Prairie Creek on a bridge, and continue past the start of the Prairie Creek Trail until you see the James Irvine Trail. The trail follows Godwood Creek through virgin redwood, Sitka spruce, Douglas-fir, and hemlock. At almost 3 miles you'll cross a bridge over the headwaters of Home Creek. Follow Home Creek down into Fern Canyon. Gold Bluffs Beach, with a pretty nice campground also worth checking out, is just beyond.

Look out for the famous banana slug (so famous, it has been proposed as the California state mollusk), bright yellow and about 6 inches long. The slugs crawl around conspicuously and like to eat all sorts of forest litter and debris. They are hermaphrodites and have penises as long as their bodies. When they mate, they impregnate each other, thus neatly opting out of the war between the sexes. Camp in August and attend the official Banana Slug Derby.

Campers looking for a little more luxury can try out one of the park's four tent cabins. Equipped with electricity and heaters, each wheelchair-accessible cabin sleeps up to six people with an outdoor tent space for up to two additional folks. Guests must bring their own bedding. Each cabin features an outdoor barbecue, a fire pit, a picnic table, and a bear locker. Pets not allowed. Reservations available at reservecalifornia.com.

Elk Prairie Campground

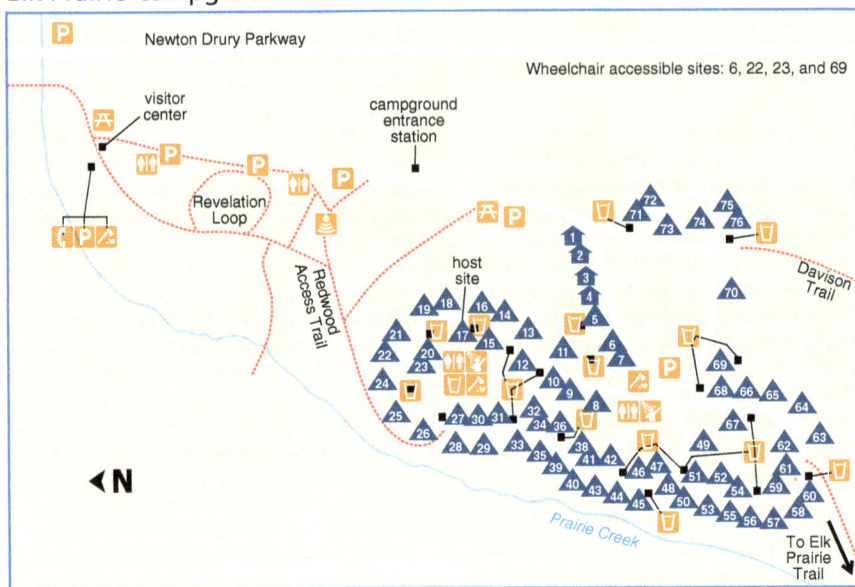

GETTING THERE

From Orick, drive 6 miles north on US 101. Go left on the Newton B. Drury Scenic Parkway and left again into Elk Prairie Campground.

GPS COORDINATES: N41° 21.539' W124° 1.802'

10

Mill Creek Campground

Beauty ★★★★★ / Privacy ★★★★★ / Spaciousness ★★★★ / Quiet ★★★ / Security ★★★★★ /
Cleanliness ★★★★★

Feels like eastern forest camping—this is the last beautiful state park to fill up on summer weekends.

Mill Creek Campground, also known as Del Norte Campground, is a pretty forest campground in a shaded stream canyon. Take away the redwoods, and this feels like eastern forest. With all the maples, it could be Pennsylvania. A mile from US 101, Mill Creek is quiet. The private campsites are backed off in their own little corners. In the summer, when everybody is on the road camping, Mill Creek fills up slowly. It is close to the Klamath River for river adventure. Crescent City is available for an emergency junk-food run—or to buy fresh fish fillets to fry back at camp. Prairie Creek Redwoods State Park is just south for trips to see the elk, or you can spend days on Gold Bluffs Beach, the most beautiful undeveloped stretch of sandy beach in California.

Del Norte Coast Redwoods State Park is huge—with more than 31,000 acres of redwoods, rhododendrons, wildflowers, tidepools, meadows, and beaches. This little corner of California is frontier. Lovely little Trinidad to the south is the last port of call for New Age California. Up here men can fix the truck, catch salmon, rig a crab trap, and run a chainsaw.

The vegetation is thick at Mill Creek Campground.

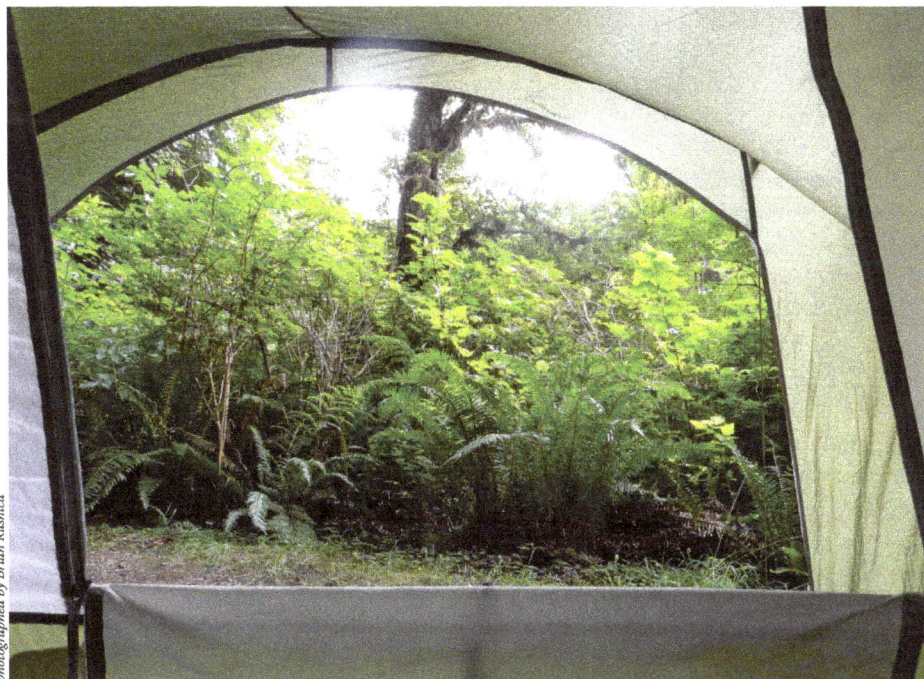

photographed by Brian Rusnica

KEY INFORMATION

LOCATION: Mill Creek Campground Road, 2 miles east of US 101, Klamath, CA 95548

OPERATED BY: Del Norte Coast Redwoods State Park and National Park Service

CONTACT: 707-465-7335; www.parks.ca.gov

OPEN: May–October

SITES: 139 sites for tents or RVs, 6 wheelchair-accessible sites

EACH SITE HAS: Picnic table, fireplace, food locker

ASSIGNMENT: First come, first served; reservations recommended

REGISTRATION: At entrance; reserve at 800-444-7275 or reservecalifornia.com

AMENITIES: Water, flush toilets, showers, firewood for sale

PARKING: At individual site

FEE: $35, $8 nonrefundable reservation fee

ELEVATION: 670'

RESTRICTIONS:

PETS: On leash only

FIRES: In fireplace

ALCOHOL: No restrictions

VEHICLES: RVs up to 31 feet, trailers up to 27 feet

OTHER: 15-day stay limit in peak season, 30-day limit in off-season; reservations recommended on summer holidays

All the women call you "Honey" and sound like they mean it. Fuel for the bellies of the folks in Del Norte County (forget pronouncing the e on Norte) is coffee, beer, and salmon jerky.

Come prepared for wet weather. Think big tent. Big tents are better if you're cooped up for a while. You get less claustrophobic and they're easier to cook in if need be. Also consider a screen house—the mosquitoes can get pesky up here as well. Plus, on a dry night, screen houses are fun to sleep in.

Mill Creek Campground is lumberjack country. Hobbs, Wall & Company once set up a private railroad called Del Norte Southern to take the logs out of Mill Creek. The redwoods grow on such steep slopes that the timber company had to build a system of railed "inclines" to the canyon and railroad below. Logs were hauled along the ridges above to an incline, where they were lowered to the canyon and railcars below.

The men did the rest of the work. They chopped the trees, limbed them, and ran the chains. It was brutal, and it gave rise to another industry—feeding 165 hungry lumberjacks down in Mill Creek three meals a day. It was serious business—each man had his seat at the table, and no one could speak until the meal was over. Mammoth quantities of meat, potatoes, canned vegetables, bread, butter, and dessert were consumed. Talk about carb- and protein-loading—these boys worked 12 hours a day, ate, and slept. Look at an old photo of the jacks—not a tubby one in the bunch—thin as rails and strong as oxen. On Saturday night they left for the bars and cathouses of Crescent City, returning to Mill Creek Canyon on Monday morning to work. There were kids in the canyon, too, and a schoolteacher to educate them. She lived in a log cabin with a drafty roof and rode the incline down to the camp every day to teach.

Hike the Trestle Trail loop along the bed of the old Hobbs, Wall & Company logging railroad that ran beside Mill Creek. Find the trailhead just northeast of the bridge between Cascara (campsites 73–125) and Red Alder Campground (campsites 1–72). The trail heads up the hillside past big stumps and maples (the alders and maples show rich color in the fall). Cross a wooden bridge and walk along the old railbed. See how the second-growth redwoods have circled the stumps of the trees cut by the company. Half a mile down the railbed, past another bridge, look for what's left of the trestle. Stay on the trail, bearing right until you come down into Red Alder Loop by campsite 7. The whole trip is a little more than a mile.

Other trails out of Mill Creek are the Hobbs Wall Trail, the Mill Creek Trail, the Alder Basin Trail, and the Saddler Skyline Trail. Hike the steep Damnation Creek Trail down to the little beach with the sea stacks and tidepools, if it's open. A structural failure to the footbridge 1.75 miles from the trailhead has kept hikers from reaching the beach but still provides access to the Coastal Trail. A shorter tidepool walk is the Enderts Beach Trail at the end of Enderts Beach Road. Find the road just south of Crescent City where Humboldt Road goes north. Drive out to Requa (once a Yurok Indian village), and hike north from the end of the road.

Crescent City is the closest supply source. Check out the Del Norte County Historical Society Museum (call 707-464-3922 for hours) or the Battery Point Lighthouse. No stranger to mishap, Crescent City was hit by a tsunami, caused by the Alaskan earthquake in 1964, that killed 14 and destroyed the downtown. And a few miles offshore, the steamer *Brother Jonathan* hit a reef and 200 passengers drowned. Win some, lose some, I guess. This is a big-shouldered frontier town.

Mill Creek Campground

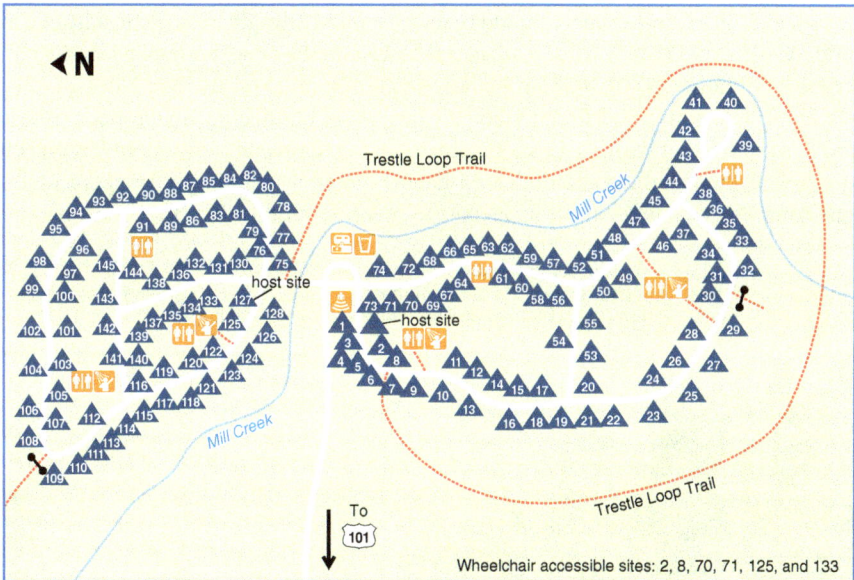

Wheelchair accessible sites: 2, 8, 70, 71, 125, and 133

GETTING THERE

From Crescent City, drive 6.5 miles south on US 101. The entrance to Mill Creek Campground is on the left. The campground is a little over 2 miles east of US 101 on the access road—look for a sign that reads DEL NORTE CAMPGROUND.

GPS COORDINATES: N41° 42.018' W124° 5.821'

11

Jedediah Smith Redwoods State Park Campgrounds

Beauty ★★★★★ / Privacy ★★★ / Spaciousness ★★★ / Quiet ★★★ / Security ★★★★★ / Cleanliness ★★★★

The northernmost of California's beautiful Redwoods State Parks—and the sun shines through the summer fog.

Jedediah Smith Redwoods State Park is gorgeous. Not only does the Smith River run by the campground for unparalleled fishing, canoeing, kayaking, and swimming, but the hiking is also great. The wild Smith River National Recreation Area is next door, and the summer weather is usually nice and sunny. Jedediah Smith Campground is fortuitously far enough east to escape the cool summer fog that plagues other state parks in redwood country. Hallelujah! The kids can paddle happily around in the river (old sneakers or water shoes of some sort are a must) while Dad sits in his lawn chair by the river and casts for trout. Meanwhile, the rays of sun will stream through the crowns of the high redwoods and splash on the ground.

Jedediah Smith Campground should really be named Sitragitum or Tcunsultum Campground for either of the two Tolowa villages that were in the area; namesake Jedediah Smith was here less than a day in 1828 on his way to getting most of his men killed in Oregon. The famous Bible-toting pathfinder made the mistake of humiliating an Umpqua tribesman whom he suspected of stealing an ax. Big mistake. Two days later, a hundred Umpqua warriors attacked and killed 16 of Smith's long-haired and buckskin-fringed trappers. Only two fought their way to safety. Smith happened to be off scouting when the attack happened,

The Smith River is the largest river system in California that flows freely along its entire course. It is a prime spot for summer swimming and fishing and for whitewater kayaking in the winter and spring.

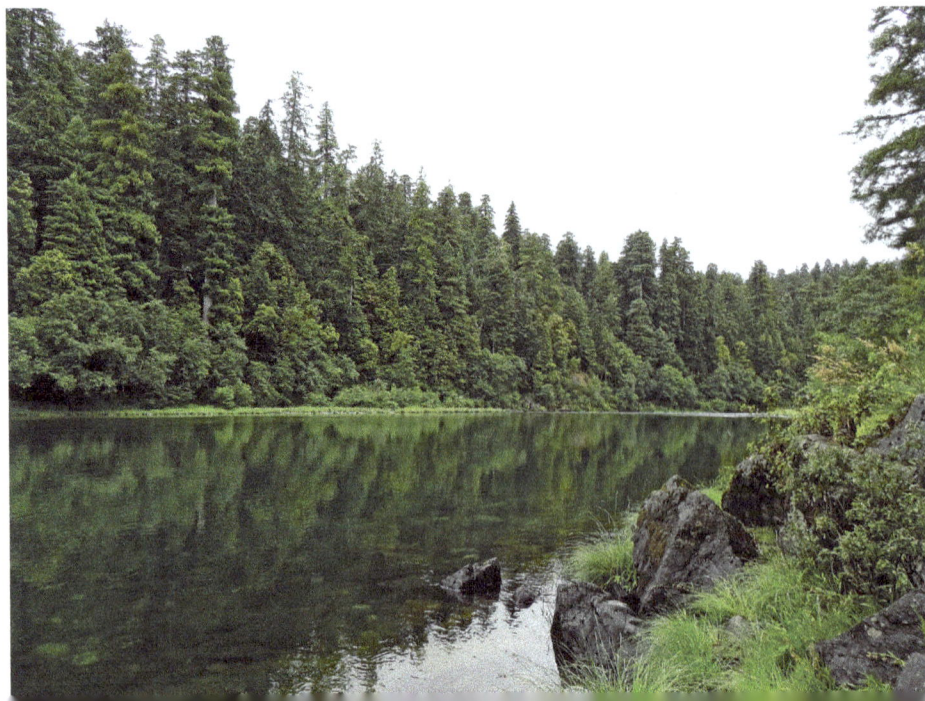

photographed by Jeff Skrentny 2014

KEY INFORMATION

LOCATION: 1461 US 199, Crescent City, CA 95531

OPERATED BY: Jedediah Smith Redwoods State Park and National Park Service

CONTACT: Camping kiosk 707-458-3018; Jedediah Smith Visitor Center (closed winters) 707-458-3496; Hiouchi Visitor Center (year-round) 707-458-3294; www.parks.ca.gov

OPEN: Year-round

SITES: 86 sites for tents or RVs, 4 cabins (wheelchair accessible)

EACH SITE HAS: Picnic table, fireplace, food locker

ASSIGNMENT: First come, first served; reservations recommended

REGISTRATION: By entrance; reserve at 800-444-7275 or reservecalifornia.com

AMENITIES: Water, flush toilets, showers, firewood for sale, wheelchair-accessible sites

PARKING: At individual site

FEE: $35, $8 nonrefundable reservation fee

ELEVATION: 150'

RESTRICTIONS:

PETS: Leashed dogs allowed in campground, not on trails

FIRES: In fireplace

ALCOHOL: No restrictions

VEHICLES: RVs and trailers up to 35 feet

OTHER: Reservations recommended on holidays and summer weekends; 15-day stay limit (3 days for hike-and-bike sites)

---

and he learned the news from one of the survivors. Smith explored on—finally losing his hair a few years later to some Comanche by a water hole on the Arkansas River.

Most of the good hiking from Jedediah Smith Campground is across the Smith River. During the summer, there is a footbridge across the river to connect with the Hiouchi Trail. The footbridge is by the winter boat launch between campsites 84 and 86. The rest of the year, prepare to get your feet wet. Remember, it's hard walking on all that river rock in your bare feet, so bring water shoes. After crossing the summer bridge or wading the river, go left for the Mill Creek Trail. The trail follows Mill Creek southeast to Howland Road and the Boy Scout Tree Road. Go right for the Simpson-Reed Discovery Trail and the Hatton Loop, which are must-see excursions. (To access them by car, exit the campground and drive 2 miles west on US 199.)

Across the highway from the Hatton Loop, the Simpson-Reed Discovery Trail is wonderfully done. Taking only about half an hour to make the loop, I learned all kinds of things about the coastal redwoods and the plants that live around them—such as how to identify the redwood sorrel, with its purple undersides and pink flowers, and why hemlock stands on its roots. Called the octopus tree, hemlock has seeds that germinate on decaying redwood logs. Its roots straddle the logs, which finally rot away, leaving the hemlock roots looking like wooden legs. I also learned that the huge redwoods come from tiny seeds—a pound of redwood seeds would start a hundred thousand trees.

Want to keep your gear to a minimum? Skip the tent and enjoy one of the park's four newly added wheelchair-accessible tent cabins, reservable at reservecalifornia.com. If you tire of the bustle of Jedediah Smith Campground, head down to Big Flat Campground off South Fork Road for some real peace and quiet. Big Flat is in the Smith River National Recreation Area, an amazing 305,337-acre hunk of wilderness in the Six River National Forest. The campground has 28 sites but no potable water. Sites cost $8 per night. To reach Big Flat

Campground, turn south on South Fork Road. Turn left after crossing the second bridge, and travel 12 miles on South Fork Road to French Hill Road. Turn left on French Hill Road and go 100 feet to the Big Flat Campground entrance on the left.

The drive south on South Fork Road is sublime. The Smith River, the last wild, undammed river in California, runs through granite gorges, through rapids, and down into deep pools. All along the road are parking spots where you can leave the car and hike down to the river. (This is fine bicycling.) Most of the trails from the parking spots head for the best steelhead bank fishing.

The nearest supply location from Jedediah Smith Campground is Hiouchi, a few hundred yards east. Hiouchi has a gas station, a small market, a café, and a decent RV park with a grass field to camp on if Jedediah Smith is packed in.

If you tire of camp grub, head down to Crescent City to the Harbor View Grotto restaurant on Starfish Way, or try the restaurant at the Ship Ashore Resort up in Smith River, just off US 101. Eat great seafood and look out over the Smith River estuary. Life can't get any better.

Jedediah Smith Redwoods State Park Campground

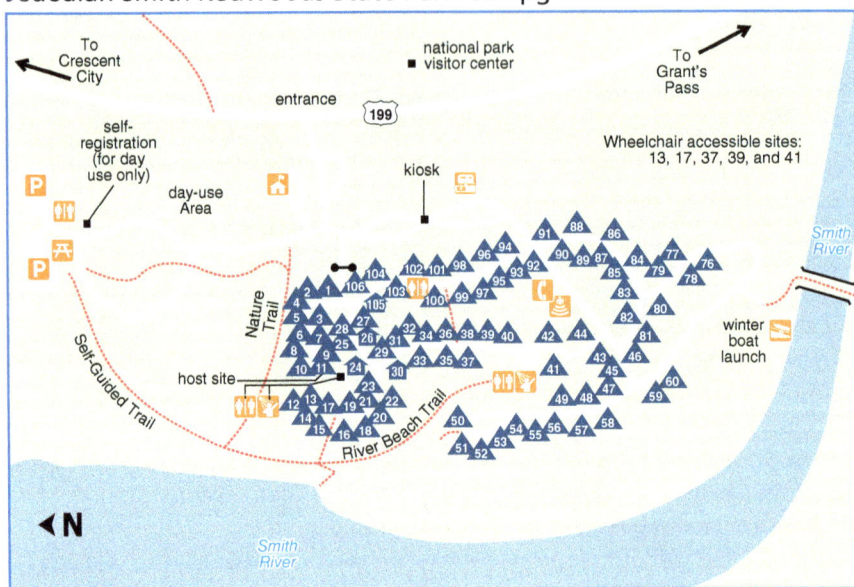

GETTING THERE

From US 101 in Crescent City, go 3.9 miles east to Exit 794 (US 199 toward Grants Pass). Continue on US 199 for 4.4 miles. The Jedediah Smith Campground is on your right before you get to Hiouchi.

GPS COORDINATES: N41° 47.892' W124° 5.045'

WINE COUNTRY

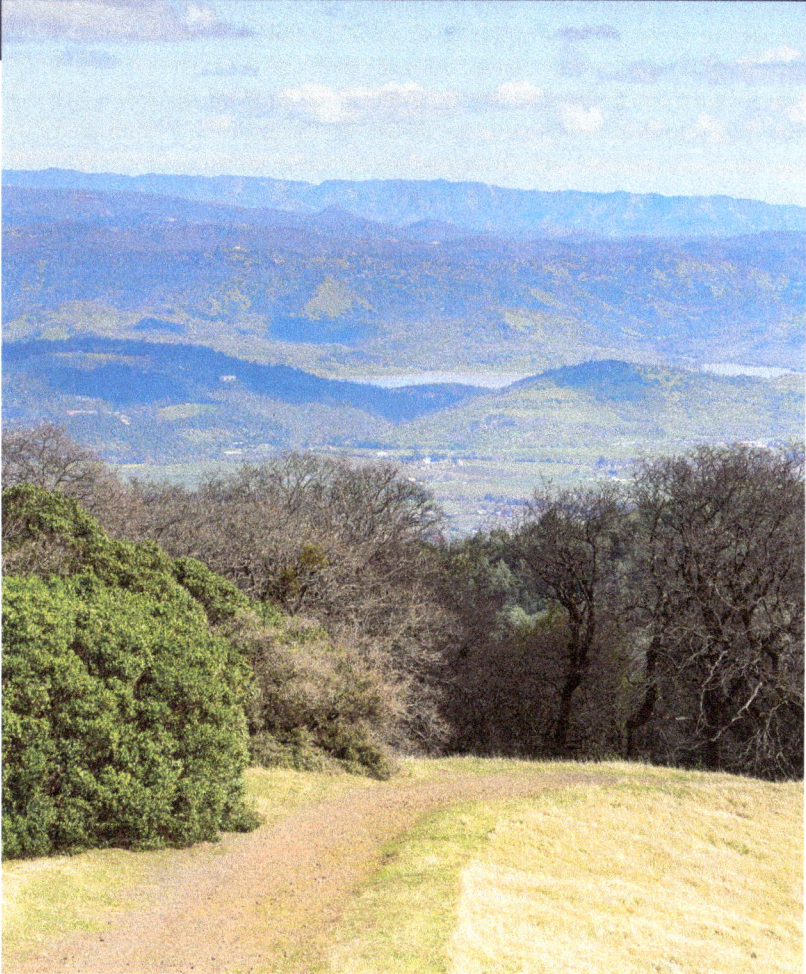

Hiking at Sugarloaf Ridge does require sunscreen, but the payoff is spectacular views of beautiful rolling hills for miles and miles *(see page 52)*.

12

⛺ Sugarloaf Ridge State Park Campgrounds

Beauty ★★★★ / Privacy ★★★ / Spaciousness ★★★★ / Quiet ★★★★ / Security ★★★★ / Cleanliness ★★★★★

Come for the wine, stay for the stars.

Say "Sonoma County" and the first thought that comes to mind probably isn't camping. With more than 400 wineries and 60,000 acres of some of the world's best-producing vineyards, the region's primary draw is to the tasting crowd. But anyone who has spent a night at Sugarloaf Ridge State Park Campground might come back for more than just the Pinot.

From Kenwood—which may look like something on a map but is actually little more than a post office, a four-aisle grocery store, and, of course, about a dozen wineries—take Adobe Canyon Road east into the Mayacama Mountains. The winding road parallels Sonoma Creek as it trickles and splashes, at one point over a 25-foot waterfall, on its way to the San Francisco Bay 33 miles from where it began. At road's end, you'll come to Sugarloaf Ridge Campground—a 47-site oasis of bucolic beauty nestled into the mountains' rolling hillsides.

From the entrance station, you can almost see the entire loop. Bordered by Sonoma Creek on the north and a hillside forest on the south, the campsites form a long ring around a large meadow in the middle. Camp along the creek, under the trees, or, especially if you have little ones who like to race around campground loops on their two-wheelers, at the far end of the loop, which has its own miniloop. Set up the camp chairs and watch the sunset turn the hills a thousand shades of pink.

Site 25 sits adjacent to the Creekside Nature Trail and is prime camping at Sugarloaf Ridge. You might even hear the gobble, gobble of a wild turkey or two.

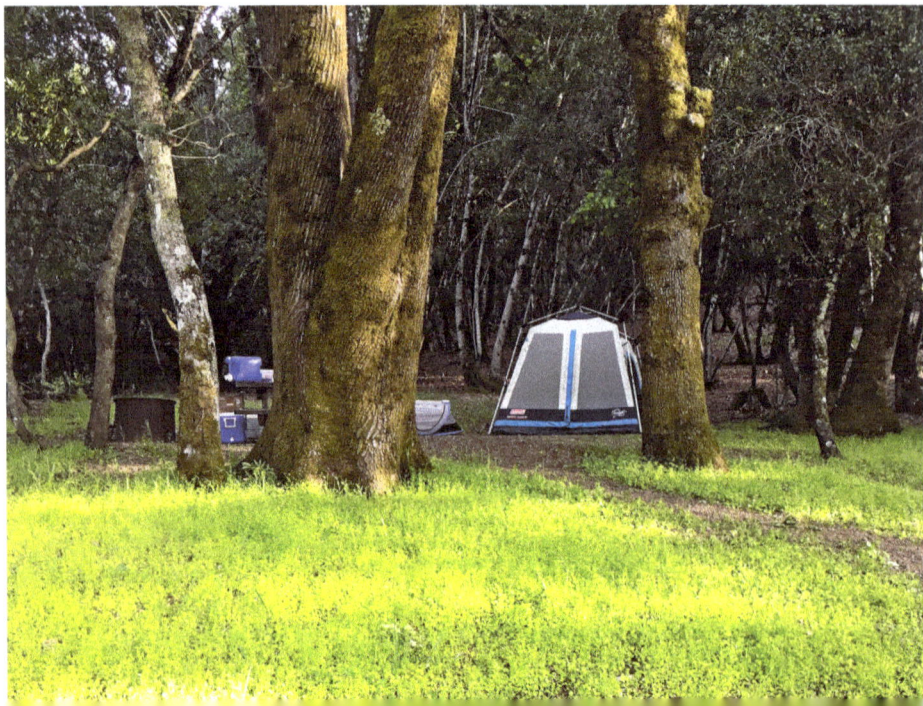

KEY INFORMATION

LOCATION: 2605 Adobe Canyon Road, Kenwood, CA 95452

OPERATED BY: Team Sugarloaf, a nonprofit consortium of Sonoma Ecology Center; United Camps, Conferences and Retreats; Sonoma County Trails Council; Robert Ferguson Observatory; and Valley of the Moon Natural History Association

CONTACT: 707-833-5712; www.parks.ca.gov; sugarloafpark.org

OPEN: Year-round

SITES: 45 total: 2 wheelchair-accessible sites, 1 group site

EACH SITE HAS: Food locker at some sites, fire pit, picnic table

ASSIGNMENT: Site specific; 10 walk-up sites are nonreservable

REGISTRATION: At park entrance; reserve at 800-444-7275 or reservecalifornia.com

AMENITIES: Hot showers, flush toilets, amphitheater, firewood for sale

PARKING: 1 car/site, overflow available

FEE: $35, $8 nonrefundable reservation fee, $8 extra vehicle

ELEVATION: 1,200'

RESTRICTIONS:

PETS: Allowed on leash, not on trails

FIRES: In pit only

ALCOHOL: No alcohol

VEHICLES: Trailers 24 feet, RV 27 feet

Wherever you pitch your tent, the camping is peaceful. The park maintains an alcohol-free policy. That doesn't mean rangers are searching bags and locking up your Sonoma Highway souvenirs until you check out; it just sends the message that this is a family-friendly campground and they want to keep it that way.

There's plenty to do here. Team Sugarloaf keeps a busy calendar, with events almost every weekend year-round. Yoga hikes are popular, as are the wildflower hikes at peak season in April, and, of course, the monthly star parties.

Yes, you read that right. The park is home to the Robert Ferguson Observatory, which prides itself on being the largest observatory in the Western United States open to the public, and for good reason: the on-site 40-inch telescope was designed and built completely by volunteers. Check the website, rfo.org, to see if your planned visit lines up with one of the monthly star parties. If not, you can either rent the observatory for you and up to 50 friends (check website for details) or show up on a Monday night for a weekly astronomy lesson (rfo.org/classes.html). Keep in mind these classes are usually geared not to the general public but to those with a serious interest in astronomy.

If you just can't get enough space travel, you can take the experience to the trail. Observatory volunteers created a 4.5-mile round-trip hike called the Planet Walk to demonstrate the vastness of the solar system. Each planet marker shows its relative size and distance from neighboring planets. After the long walk in the blazing sun, you might rethink your decision to go all the way to Pluto, which was after all reclassified as a dwarf planet, but it definitely provides perspective.

Much of the hiking at Sugarloaf requires copious amounts of sunscreen. If it's shade you seek, stick to the Canyon Trail, which descends from just downhill of the park entrance alongside Sonoma Creek, and get a look at the splashy 25-foot falls. Make it super family-friendly and set a shuttle car about a mile down the road so nobody needs to climb the 400 feet back up the hill. Find more shady-ish hiking on the Godspeed Trail to Hood

Mountain, but don't expect a view. If you're going for a grand vista, you'll need to brace yourself for the sunrays, keep a keen eye out for rattlesnakes, and take a trail up to Bald Mountain (2,972'). There are several ways to get there: The most direct follows an old paved road. The shadiest way is a combination of the Red Mountain, Vista, and Headwaters Trails, but you'll still need to walk the road at least a little. You won't be disappointed. From the top there's a spectacular 360-degree view—the Sierra Nevada to the San Francisco Bay, Mount Tamalpais to Mount Saint Helena—as lovely or more so than the finest glass of vino.

Note: Sugarloaf Ridge State Park incurred damage to its water system, forests, and some trails due to the 2017 Nuns Fire. As of publication, campground officials expect the park and campground to be fully operational by summer 2018.

Sugarloaf Ridge State Park Campground

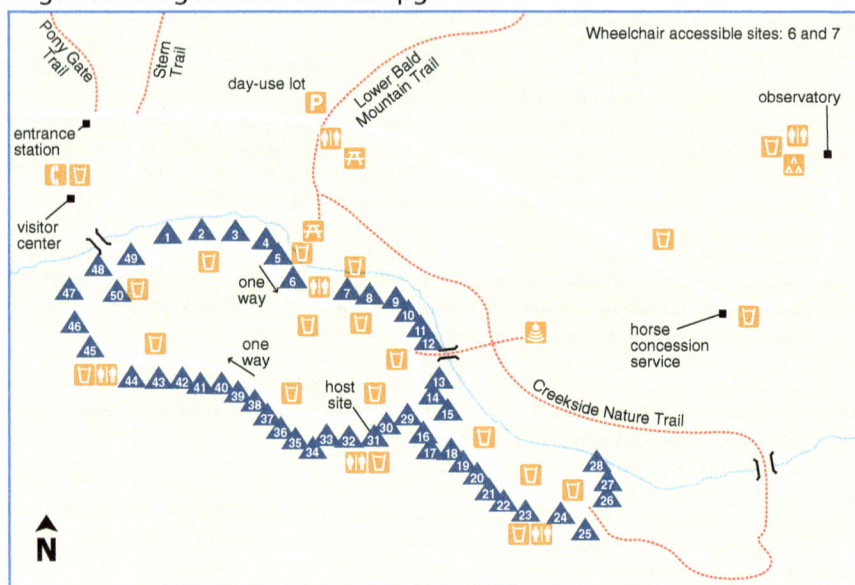

GETTING THERE

From San Francisco, follow US 101 north about 50 miles to Santa Rosa. Take Exit 488B for CA 12. At the end of the exit ramp, take a left onto Farmers Lane, and go 1 mile. Turn right onto CA 12, and head east 8.4 miles. Turn left onto Adobe Canyon Road. Follow the road 2 miles to the entrance station.

GPS COORDINATES: N38° 26.272' W122° 30.859'

13

⛺ Hendy Woods State Park Campgrounds

Beauty ★★★ / Privacy ★★★ / Spaciousness ★★★★ / Quiet ★★★ / Security ★★★ / Cleanliness ★★★★

OTHER: Fishing is not allowed on the Navarro River inside the park

A park of the people, by the people, and for the people

In a parallel universe, there would be no Hendy Woods State Park Campgrounds. In 2011, when 70 California state parks were on the chopping block, Hendy Woods was scheduled for closure in 2012. At that time, the park spent approximately $200,000 more each year on operating costs than it brought in. Less than 50,000 people visited the 816-acre park, making it a little too quiet for legislators trying to balance budgets. Fortunately, something about the silent, ancient coast redwoods defies price tags.

The history of Hendy's twin old-growth groves, 20-acre Little Hendy and 80-acre Big Hendy, is a chain of near misses and passionate protection. The groves' first official known owner was Joshua Hendy, a businessman who moved to California from Texas during the gold rush and built a large sawmill on the Navarro River. Hendy's trees held a special place in his heart, and when he died in 1891 he willed them to his nephew Samuel Hendy to protect them. But times got tough for Samuel, and the broke chap sold the groves to the Pacific

Just a short leg-stretcher from each of the Hendy Woods campgrounds, Little Hendy Grove exudes a mystical energy you have to experience in person.

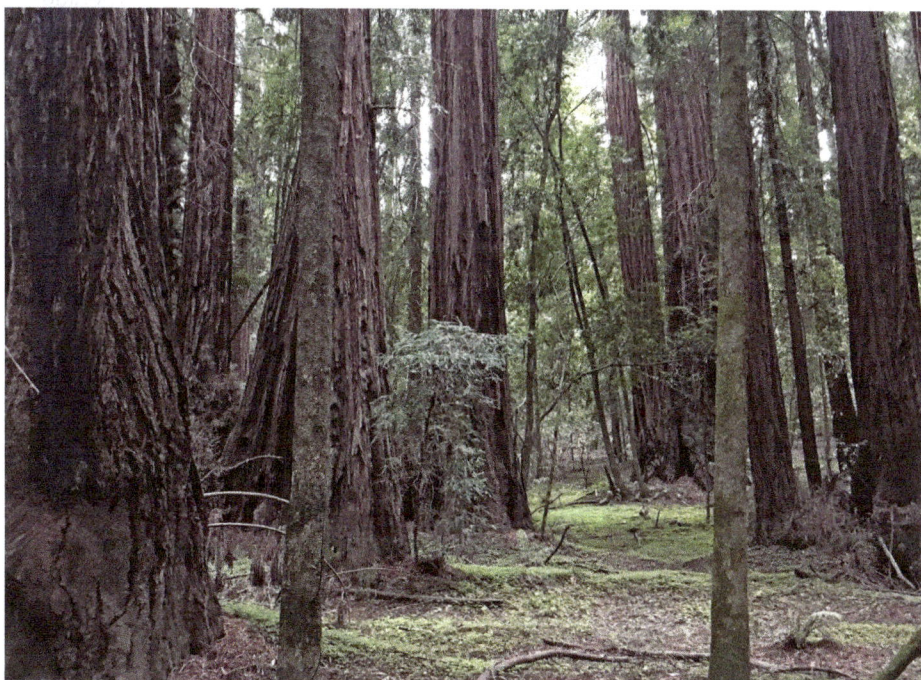

KEY INFORMATION

LOCATION: 18599 Philo Greenwood Road, Philo, CA 95466

OPERATED BY: Hendy Woods State Park

CONTACT: 707-895-3141; www.parks.ca.gov

OPEN: Year-round (reservable May–September)

SITES: 77 total: 2 hike-and-bike sites, 5 wheelchair-accessible sites, 4 tent cabins

EACH SITE HAS: Small food locker, fire pit, picnic table

ASSIGNMENT: Site specific

REGISTRATION: At park entrance; reserve at 800-444-7275 or reservecalifornia.com

AMENITIES: Hot showers, flush toilets, firewood for sale

PARKING: 2 cars/site, overflow available

FEE: $45 peak season, $40 all other times, $70 cabins, $10 hike-and-bike sites, $10 extra vehicle

ELEVATION: 1,200'

RESTRICTIONS:

PETS: Allowed in day-use area, campground, and fire road; must be on leash

FIRES: In pit only; no gathering of firewood

ALCOHOL: No restrictions

VEHICLES: RVs and trailers up to 35 feet

Coast Lumber Company a few years later. The groves changed hands twice more, each time to a different logging company, but were spared the blade. Then in 1948, a band of passionate women belonging to the Anderson Valley Unity Club grew skeptical of sleeping with the enemy and decided to pressure the state to purchase the groves and develop a park to ensure their protection.

Their work paid off. The state purchased the groves from the Masonite Corporation in 1958 and officially dedicated the park and campground five years later, providing the largest river access in Anderson Valley. In 2011, that protection came under scrutiny as state legislators contemplated Hendy's closure. Concerned citizens banded together. A young group of activists enlisted help from the Occupy movement, most popular for its protests on Wall Street. They protested, sent letters, wrote articles, and held teach-ins arguing that the groves' critical role in maintaining a healthy Navarro River was too great to overlook.

Once again, the hard work paid off. With help from the newly formed Hendy Woods Community, the state park remains open today. Come here to camp in the trees at one of the 92 spacious sites that sit underneath a dense forest of madrone, Douglas-fir, and California laurel. with a smattering of solo coast giants decorating a few sites. Both groves are an easy walk from the campground, and each exudes a mysterious, magical energy that you'll have to feel to truly understand. Hike to the Hendy Hut from your site, a lean-to of redwood planks against a stump that housed Russian immigrant Petrov Zailenko for 18 years in the 1960 and '70s.

While the trees, some 300 feet tall and more than 1,000 years old, certainly take center stage, there's more to do than just wander the woods. Picnicking along the 3.3 miles of river frontage in the park is popular. This gentle section also lends itself to floaters, so bring your own craft and take out at the Philo-Greenwood bridge. Anderson Valley is well known as a less expensive and arguably more intimate destination for wine tasting, with dozens of wineries within 10 miles of the park. Anderson Valley Brewing Company is headquartered just a few miles south of the park in Boonville.

Grapes and hops aren't the only agricultural stars of this lush, fertile valley; this is apple country too. On the eastern edge of the park, rows of orchards border Little Hendy Grove. Less than a mile from the park's entrance, you can buy jams, apple butters, juice, and cider, as well as a seasonal selection of greens and farm-fresh eggs when available at the Philo Apple Farm stand. Another farm-to-table highlight is the Pennyroyal goat cheese farm in Boonville, which offers family-friendly tours of its biodynamic sheep farm and, of course, a wine and cheese tasting.

Don't expect too much else to eat on the road, though. Restaurants are few and far between, and groceries are limited to a small store in Boonville. Stock up on camp food before you leave home, and come ready to bask in the glory of the giants.

Hendy Woods State Park Campgrounds

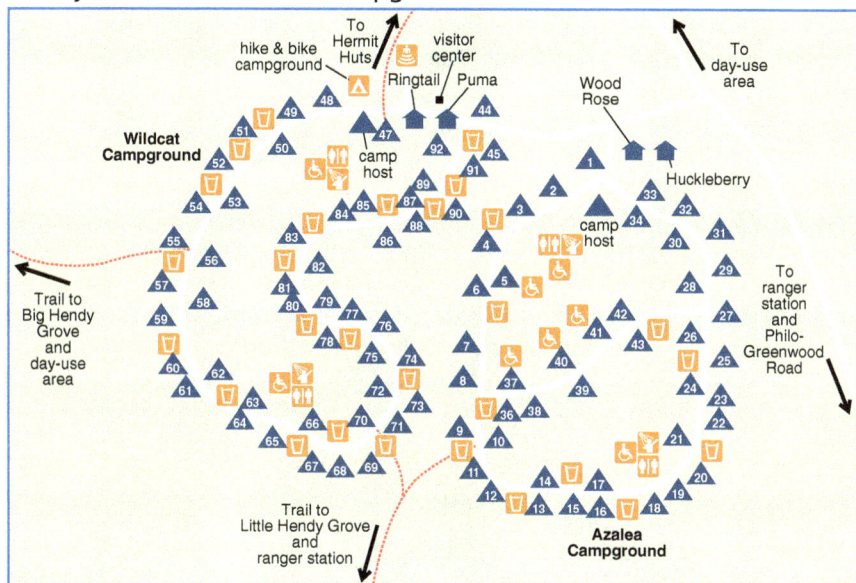

GETTING THERE

From Santa Rosa, follow US 101 north 32.5 miles to Exit 522 (CA 128 Fort Bragg/Mendocino). Turn left onto CA 128, and head west 35 miles. Turn left onto Greenwood Road/Philo Greenwood Road. In 0.6 mile cross the Navarro River and turn left into Hendy Woods State Park.

GPS COORDINATES: N39° 4.188' W123° 28.254'

14

Albee Creek Campground

Beauty ★★★★★ / Privacy ★★★ / Spaciousness ★★★★ / Quiet ★★★ / Security ★★★★★ /
Cleanliness ★★★★

Come out of the big trees and into the sunshine at this pretty little spot.

Drive 5 miles off US 101 on Mattole Road through incredible stands of redwoods (use daytime headlights) and come to Albee Creek Campground 0.3 mile up an access road on the right. This beautiful campground is framed by Albee Creek on the east and Bull Creek on the south—most of the campsites nestle at the base of a forested hillside to the north. This is nice open camping for folks who don't want the "darkness at noon" aspect of the redwood forest. Down below on the little prairie is an old fruit orchard planted by John Albee, who carried mail into Bull Valley in the old days, before the forest became Humboldt Redwoods State Park.

From Albee Campground, catch the Big Trees–Albee Creek Loop Trail. This is a 2.5-mile round-trip hike that follows Albee Creek east as it meanders just south of Mattole Road through the Rockefeller Forest, the world's largest grove of old-growth redwoods. The average age of these trees falls between 500 and 1,200 years, with the oldest-known tree at 2,200 years old. Many measure more than 300 feet high, with some topping 360 feet. Hike under these trees among the calypso orchids, fetid adder's-tongues, and redwood sorrel, and think about what the trees meant to the American Indians in this region. They used them to make dugout canoes, plank and bark houses, and furniture. The shredded inner bark was made into women's skirts.

Albee Creek Campground is inside Humboldt Redwoods State Park along the Avenue of the Giants.

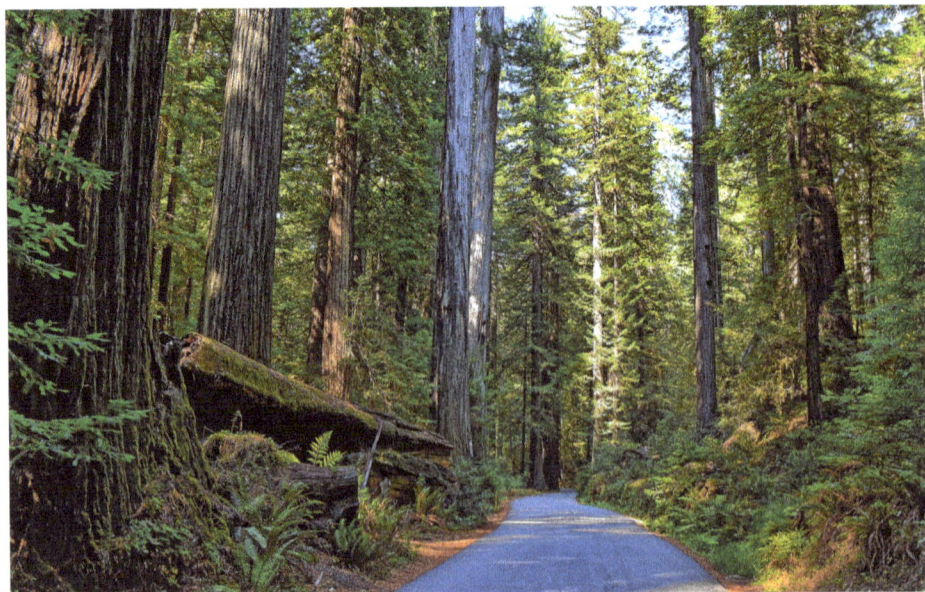

photographed by Kirt Edblom

KEY INFORMATION

LOCATION: 17119 Avenue of the Giants, Weott, CA 95571

OPERATED BY: Humboldt Redwoods State Park

CONTACT: Camping kiosk 707-946-2472; headquarters 707-946-2409; www.parks.ca.gov or humboldtredwoods.org

OPEN: May–mid-October

SITES: 22 sites for tents, 18 sites for tents or RVs

EACH SITE HAS: Picnic table, fireplace, food locker

ASSIGNMENT: Reservations 2 days–7 months in advance; reservations recommended; otherwise, first come, first served

REGISTRATION: At entrance; reserve at 800-444-7275 or reservecalifornia.com

AMENITIES: Water, flush toilets, coin-operated showers, firewood for sale, wheelchair-accessible sites

PARKING: At individual site; $8 extra vehicle

FEE: $35, $8 nonrefundable reservation fee

ELEVATION: 320'

RESTRICTIONS:

PETS: Dogs on leash only, in campground

FIRES: In fireplace

ALCOHOL: No restrictions

VEHICLES: RVs up to 24 feet

OTHER: 7-day stay limit

The first strangers to see the redwoods were the Chinese more than 2,000 years ago. Accounts tell of a junk captain, Hee-li, who followed his compass in the direction he thought was east (what did he think when he saw the sun setting in the east instead of the west?). Four months later he landed in a place with wonderful weather and gigantic trees with thick, reddish bark. Hee-li checked out his compass and found a small cockroach wedged under the needle. Upon removal of the cockroach, the needle swung around, and Hee-li sailed back home to China.

Next came the Spanish missionaries, who saw the redwoods near Monterey and cut them for roof beams in the missions. They soon realized that Palo Colorado had wonderful properties. Father Junipero Serra had his coffin made of redwood, and it was in perfect condition when it was exhumed a century later.

Then Dr. Josiah Gregg and a group of forty-niners came through these parts and discovered Humboldt Bay (which he named after his hero, Alexander von Humboldt, a 19th-century German scientist, naturalist, and geographer). Gold was discovered on the Trinity and the Klamath Rivers. Forty-niners flooded north in 1850, and Humboldt County, with its wonderful bay and bountiful redwoods, was on its way to being the most populated region on the northern coast.

A big draw in the park is the Eel River, with springtime canoeing and the wildflower bloom. Hike down along the Eel, and pick up the River Trail where the Big Trees–Albee Creek Trail loops back around near the Rockefeller Loop. From here, the River Trail heads down the west side of the Eel to the Children's Forest, where a stone marker records the names of local children who died in the early 1900s. The fire-hollowed trees here once were goose pens. The round-trip just tops 5 miles.

As tame as Albee Creek, Bull Creek, and the Eel River look in the summer and fall, think twice: In 1955 and 1964 there were monster floods here. On the way from Garberville on US 101, look for the markers far above the highway that record the level of the raging water at the height of the flood. In 1955, near Albee Campground, Bull Creek raged through the town of Bull Creek, taking out 35 houses and the cemetery. Later, coffins were found in the branches of redwoods in the Rockefeller Forest.

Drive west on Mattole Road to Panther Gap (2,477') and look over the watershed that these creeks and river service. When excessive logging cleared away the trees, there was nothing to stop the rain running off the slopes. The locals are thus caught on the horns of a dilemma: many work for the lumber companies, but none of them want to see their houses swept away when the floods come.

Continue over Panther Gap down to the picturesque little hamlet of Honeydew (named for the sweet-tasting aphid dew beneath cottonwoods down by the river). There's good fishing on the Mattole River between Honeydew and Petrolia.

Humboldt Redwoods State Park has huge trees and huge mosquitoes in the late spring and summer—prepare! If you're planning a visit in May or October, call ahead to check for road closures due to two annual marathons in the spring and fall.

Albee Creek Campground

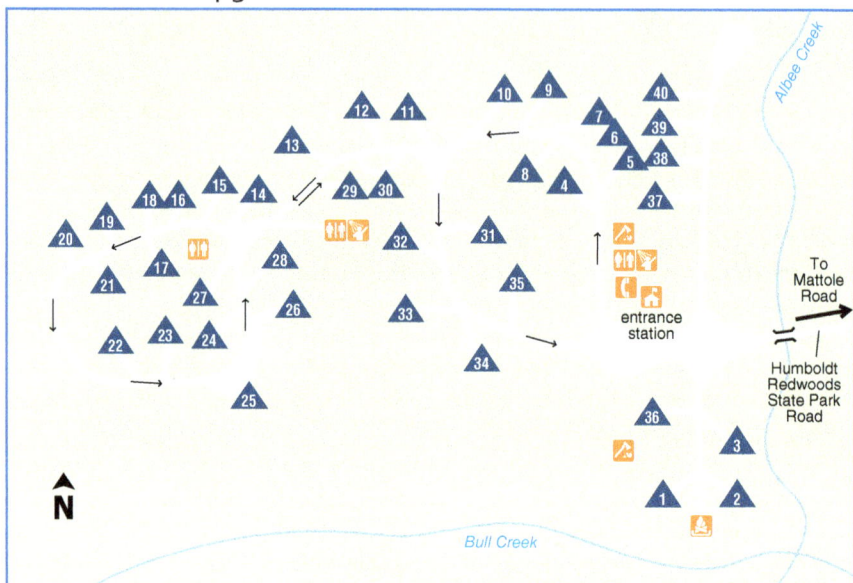

GETTING THERE

From Weott, north of Garberville, drive 2 miles north to Mattole Road, then drive west 5 miles to the Albee Creek Campground entrance on the right. Go 0.3 mile up the access road to the campground.

GPS COORDINATES: N40° 21.170' W124° 0.563'

SHASTA-TRINITY

Lewiston Lake's placid waters are a paddler's dream *(see page 62)*. This 5-mile-long lake has a strict speed limit of 10 miles per hour for motorboats, making it ideal for angling kayakers and canoeists.

15

Mary Smith and Cooper Gulch Campgrounds

Beauty ★★★★ / Privacy ★★★ / Spaciousness ★★★ / Quiet ★★★★ / Security ★★★★ / Cleanliness ★★★★★

Fish, paddle, or simply relax on the shores of Lewiston Lake with a view from your campsite.

If you're a die-hard lake lover but reservoir ring has you down, head up to Lewiston Lake—the last reservoir on the Trinity River before the river flows wild and free to the Pacific. Lewiston, with its clean, clear, and cool waters, is always full—even in a drought. The quiet, 750-acre lake restricts motorized boats to a speed of less than 10 miles per hour and is well stocked with rainbows, browns, and kokanee salmon. The placid waters are ideal for paddlers, and campers at Mary Smith and Cooper Gulch Campgrounds have front-door access to this aquamarine paradise.

Mary Smith is the more popular of the two campgrounds. Set off a bit farther from the road, it has a more tucked-in feeling. The campground, which has received attention from popular magazines and newspapers as one of the very best in tent camping, offers 12 campsites without the eyesore of an RV—no trailers allowed. There's just one catch: glampers. Funny word, isn't it? Glamping is camping without the backaches of sleeping on the ground, and glamping units are tent cabins that occupy campsites. The six glamping units at Mary Smith feature sturdy decks, armchairs, barbecue grills, a queen bed with fresh linens, and even a dresser drawer next to the bed. The tent cabins are waterproof (a nice option if you

Just steps from Lewiston Lake, sites at Cooper Gulch Campground are flat and nicely spaced.

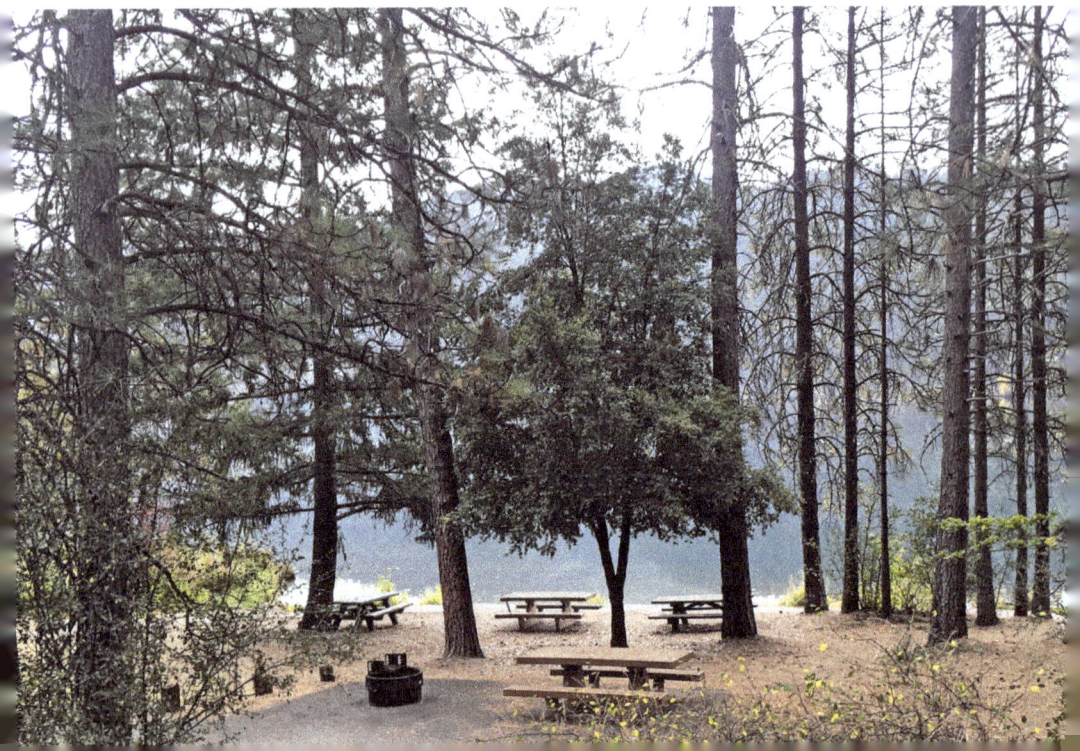

KEY INFORMATION

LOCATION: 5480 Trinity Dam Blvd., Lewiston, CA 96052

OPERATED BY: Shasta Recreation Company; Shasta-Trinity National Forest, Weaverville Ranger District

CONTACT: Weaverville Ranger Station 530-623-2121; Shasta Recreation Company 530-275-8113; www.fs.usda.gov/stnf; shastatrinitycamping.com

OPEN: May–mid-October

SITES: Mary Smith: 17 total, 11 walk-in sites, 6 glamping sites; Cooper Gulch: 5 sites

EACH SITE HAS: Picnic table, fire pit, grill

ASSIGNMENT: First come, first served; reservations available (and recommended)

REGISTRATION: At entrance; reserve at 877-444-6777 or recreation.gov

AMENITIES: Drinking water, vault and flush toilet (no showers)

PARKING: 3 parking areas access 3 different loops of the campground. All sites require at least a 25-foot walk-in.

FEE: $20, $6 extra vehicle, $85 glamping tent cabins, $9 nonrefundable reservation fee

ELEVATION: 1,902'

RESTRICTIONS:

PETS: On leash only

FIRES: In fire pit

ALCOHOL: No restrictions

VEHICLES: No RVs allowed

---

happen to get caught in a rogue storm without a sufficient rain fly), and they aren't cheap: nightly rates are about $85.

Glamping is on the rise in Northern California state parks and national forests. Oftentimes glamping units are positioned on the outer edge of a loop and are grouped together. At Mary Smith, if you're not a fan of glampers, you will need to be strategic about picking your site. The campground is divided into three groups with three parking areas (all sites are walk-in). Sites 1–9 make up the first group with a mix of traditional campsites and glamping units. Sites in this group provide the easiest access to the lake, the least privacy, and a clean bathroom with flush toilets. For more privacy, compromised lake access, and steep walk-ups, consider sites 10–14. What you sacrifice in burning calves from the steep walk-ups, you gain in views and privacy. The last group is just a couple—sites 16 and 17. These sites are truly removed from the rest. Perched up on a hill with views of the lake through the trees, each site has a rugged walk-in, and they share a vault toilet.

Three bits of advice about Mary Smith: 1. Bring a kayak, canoe, or something to paddle on the water, or plan on renting something at the marina a few miles up the road. 2. Don't worry about bringing your bike. The terrain is too hilly for a casual after-dinner pedal around camp. 3. Think twice about bringing a family with young kids or any pets—poison oak thrives here, and open spaces to play are few and far between. Family camping is a bit nicer just up the street (or trail) at Cooper Gulch. This small five-site campground offers nice, flat sites, all with a clear view of the lake. Lake access is superb. The one drawback at Cooper Gulch is the road. Trinity Dam Boulevard isn't exactly a major thoroughfare, but enough cars and trucks drive by at night with enough speed that if you're sensitive to it at all it just might drive you nuts.

To stretch your legs, there's a pretty, 1.5-mile doubletrack trail along the lakeshore that connects Mary Smith to Cooper Gulch. Actual lake access along this trail is minimal due to the steep shoreline, but it's a nice trail with pretty views, especially in late September, when the maples turn bright orange, yellow, and red. Another must-do while you're in the area

Mary Smith Campground

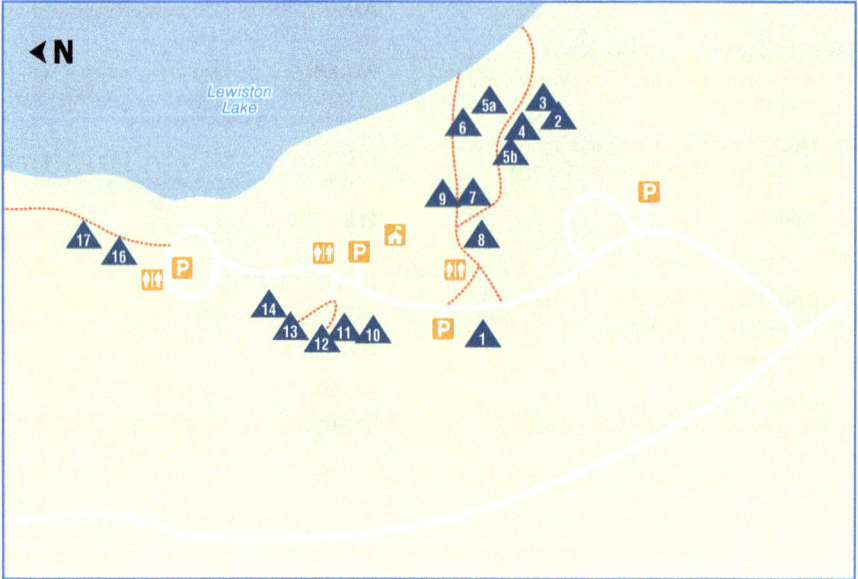

Cooper Gulch Campground

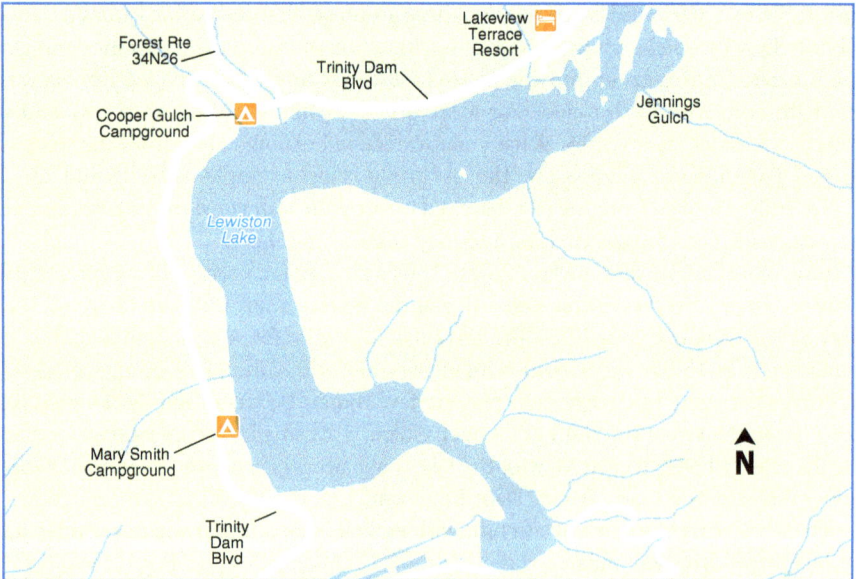

is the Trinity River Hatchery, just below the Lewiston Dam. It's open all year, but the best time to visit the hatchery is September–March, when the fish ladder is open. The hatchery raises a spring and fall run of chinook salmon, coho salmon (though recreational angling for coho in California is prohibited), and steelhead. Watch the fish jump the ladder through viewing windows at the hatchery. Visit early morning on a Monday or Thursday and you can even check out spawning operations. There's always something interesting to do or see there. The last time we visited in early October, my 4-year-old son got the chance to feed the fish in the holding ponds (a trip highlight), and we witnessed a juvenile release! After two years in a pen, hundreds of fish were swept from their home into the river. The collective joy of graduation day for these adolescent animals was palpable, as was their angst while flocks of cormorant birds eagerly awaited their chance for a feast. Visit wildlife.ca.gov/fishing/hatcheries/trinity-river for up-to-date information and event listings; there's always something fun to do there.

GETTING THERE

From Weaverville: Take CA 3 north 7 miles. Turn right on Rush Creek Road and go 9 miles. Turn left on Trinity Dam Boulevard and go 1.3 miles to Mary Smith Campground or 2.7 miles to Cooper Gulch.

GPS COORDINATES: N40° 43.741' W122° 48.396'

16

Antlers Campground

Beauty ★★★★ / Privacy ★★★★ / Spaciousness ★★★ / Quiet ★★ / Security ★★★★ /
Cleanliness ★★★★

The three Shastas—dam, lake, and volcano—are the most dominant forces in this northern country.

Not to be confused with Antlers RV Park & Campground, which is a private campground just a quarter mile down the road, Antlers Campground offers one of many opportunities for tent camping around Lake Shasta. It's a favorite of mine for its convenience, great camp host, boat ramp, clean grounds and facilities, and surprising quiet despite being within minutes of I-5.

In 1948, Shasta Dam was completed after controversy, a number of deaths, and a delay because of World War II, becoming one of the greatest civil-engineering feats in the world at that time. An arch-gravity dam, similar to the Hoover Dam, it was created using the continuous-pour concrete method.

When traveling north on I-5, refuel in Redding and stop by the Turtle Bay Exploration Park for further history on the dam and Lake Shasta region. Located beside the internationally acclaimed Sundial Bridge, the park offers information and videos on the dam's construction (among a wide variety of other interesting activities and exhibits for every age).

Shasta Dam changed the entire landscape of Northern California; created hydroelectricity and irrigation for the state; and, let us not forget, formed quite a magnificent lake. The Pit, McCloud, and Sacramento Rivers feed Lake Shasta, but only the Sacramento is released behind the 602-foot-high, 3,469-foot-long concrete wall to flow from Redding through Sacramento and eventually into San Francisco Bay.

Turtle Bay Exploration Park, about 30 minutes south in Redding, is a worthy day trip. It features dozens of themed gardens, environmental education camps, animals, the Sundial Bridge, and more.

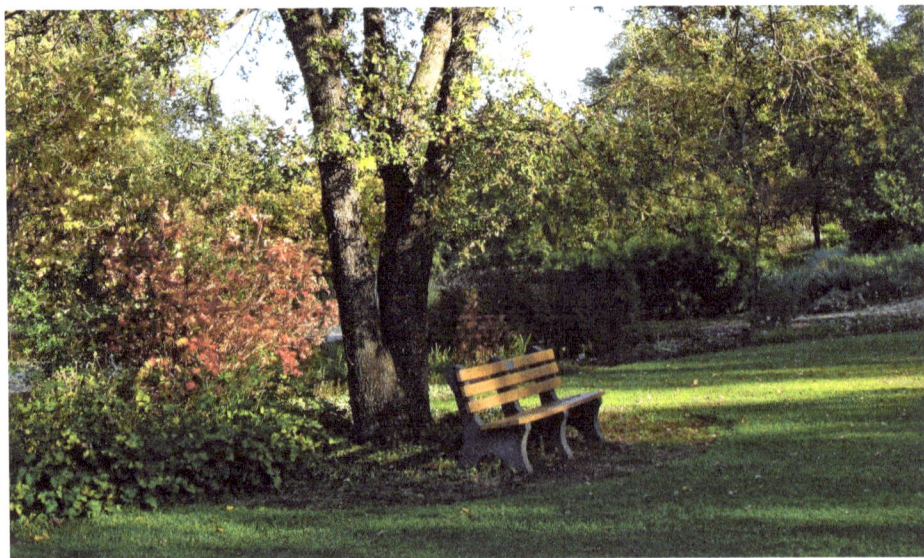

photographed by Eleanor Taniguchi

KEY INFORMATION

LOCATION: Antlers Road (Exit 702 from I-5), Lakehead, CA 96051

OPERATED BY: Shasta Recreation Company; Shasta-Trinity National Forest, Shasta Lake Ranger District

CONTACT: Shasta Lake Ranger Station 530-275-1587; Shasta Recreation Company 530-275-8113; www.fs.usda.gov/stnf; shastatrinitycamping.com

OPEN: March 1–October 31; reservations May 15–mid-September

SITES: 59

EACH SITE HAS: Picnic table, fireplace, grill, food locker

ASSIGNMENT: First come, first served; reservations available (14 not reservable)

REGISTRATION: At entrance; reserve at 877-444-6777 or recreation.gov

AMENITIES: Water, flush and vault toilets, boat launch

PARKING: At individual site

FEE: $20 single, $35 double, $6 extra vehicle

ELEVATION: 600'

RESTRICTIONS:

PETS: On leash, only 2 pets/campsite

FIRES: In fireplace

ALCOHOL: No restrictions

VEHICLES: RVs up to 40 feet

OTHER: 14-day stay limit

I've met a few people who remember the thriving mining towns that were swallowed beneath the lake's depths—517 feet at its deepest—like the town of Kennett, which once had a population of more than 10,000. Lake Shasta also entombed Wintu Indian sacred lands and burial sites, though many of these were moved.

Today, Lake Shasta is a recreation mecca. There are many exploring options available with 370 miles of shoreline. It's the largest man-made reservoir in California and often appears to be several separate lakes when you're cruising up I-5 after finally rising out of the top of the long Sacramento Valley. About 10 miles north of Redding, the highway starts hugging the mountains, and then come the sudden glimpses and views of a vast lake.

Antlers Campground is located at the tiny town of Lakehead and is much larger than it first appears. Several loops wind through the tall oaks, firs, and pines. You won't be lounging on the beach or jumping into the lake from your campsite here. The campground rests on a cliff above the lake, and depending on water levels, that cliff can be quite significant. There is lake access at the boat ramp and by half-hidden trails, but be careful. By the way, Lake Shasta doesn't have any beach areas, just plenty of smooth red earth both below and above the surface.

Don't forget the earplugs! Even if you love the sound of the train, you might not be such a big fan in the middle of the night.

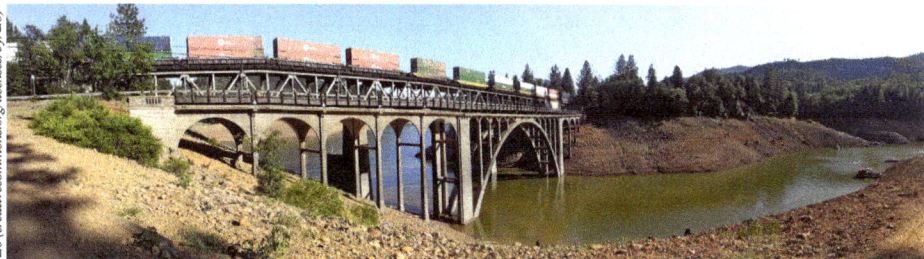

The most dramatic views are at campsites on the outside of the loop, but these sites are not for children. The inside sites are perfect for kids, and the pines and tall oaks all around provide beauty and shade from the afternoon heat—this is especially appreciated in July to early September, when the temperatures may reach the triple digits.

The contrast of color on Lake Shasta is striking, with vibrant sienna earth and deep-green forests sandwiched between the fluctuating blues of water and sky.

If you'll be boating on the lake or fishing on its edges, you should fill up the gas tank and explore the three river arms that feed Lake Shasta. There's excellent fishing here, with bass tournaments held at various times throughout the year.

The wildlife at Antlers is plentiful—boating friends often tell me they see bears and deer, among many other forest critters, along the shoreline. We spotted a bald eagle the last time we visited.

Within a 15-minute drive, you can find various other points of interest, including Shasta Caverns; Bridge Bay Marina; and Shasta Dam, which features an informative visitor center and the opportunity to walk across the dam. The three Shastas—dam, lake, and volcano—are the most dominant forces in this northern country, and they will surely satisfy water enthusiasts, mountain lovers, history buffs, or anyone searching for outdoor excitement.

Antlers Campground

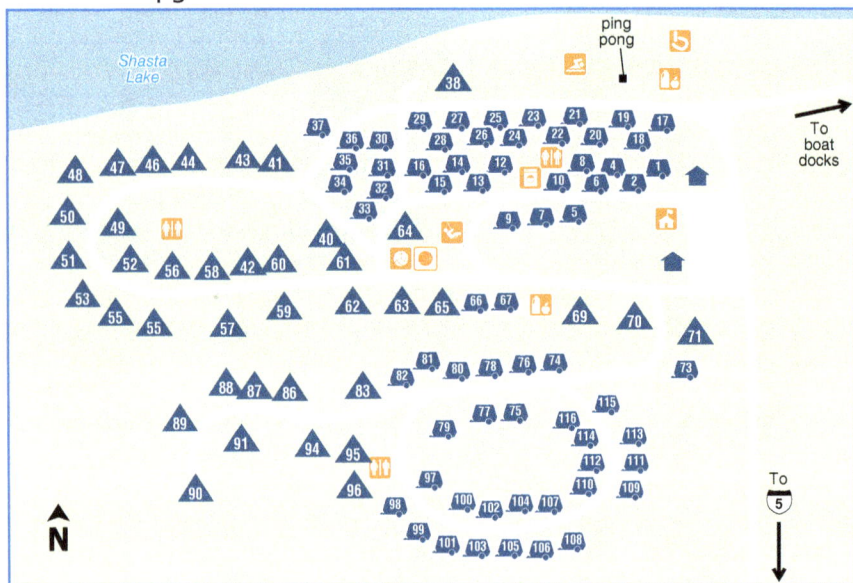

GETTING THERE

From Redding, drive 24 miles north on I-5, and take Exit 702, turning right at the end of the off-ramp. Almost immediately turn right onto Antlers Road and proceed 0.8 mile, first going south, then going north again. The campground entrance is on the right.

GPS COORDINATES: N40° 53.243' W122° 22.718'

17

Tish Tang Campground

Beauty ★★★★ / Privacy ★★★★ / Spaciousness ★★★★ / Quiet ★★★★ / Security ★★★★ / Cleanliness ★★★★

Welcome to the place where the land sticks out and touches the water, the pride of the Hoopa tribe, and the heart of the Trinity River.

Tish Tang is a campground in the Hoopa Valley Indian Reservation, surrounded by Six Rivers National Forest. The mighty Trinity River calls out the siren song here, luring campers to a rocky-banked, cool river and lulling them to sleep at night with soothing white noise.

To reach the campground, turn off CA 96 and descend a steep, sharply switchbacking paved road. As you enter the campground and bear left onto the one-way road, the first series of sites on the left back up to the forested hillside. All sites in the campground are at least partially shaded, but these offer the most tree cover. There's a group campsite on the right about halfway through the campground that offers a large, grassy open area for multiple tents and a new group site that doubles as a wedding site for couples who want to tie the knot overlooking the river. Sites on the back stretch of the road offer the easiest access to the river, but from any of the sites at Tish Tang, the Trinity is mere moments away.

There are two access paths to the river: one a trail departing between sites 25 and 27, and the other a gravel road that descends to the beach from a small parking area just outside the

The 165-mile Trinity River is an excellent place for fishing, swimming, and rafting.

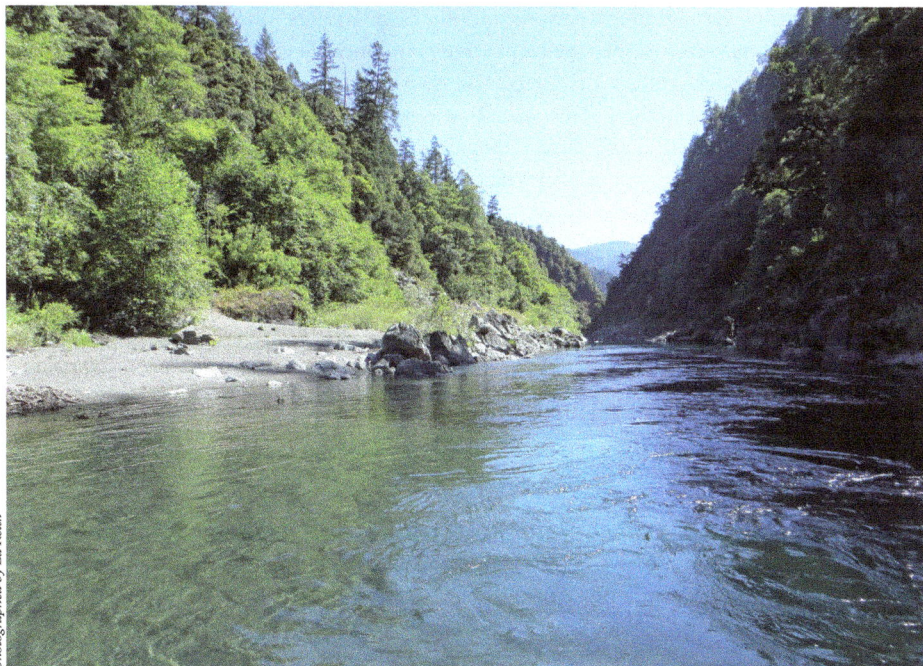

photographed by Ed Keith

KEY INFORMATION

LOCATION: CA 96, 7 miles north of CA 299, Hoopa, CA

OPERATED BY: Hoopa Valley Tribal Council

CONTACT: 707-672-6018, hoopaforestry .com/campground.html

OPEN: Year-round

SITES: 38 sites for tents and RVs up to 44 feet, 2 group sites

EACH SITE HAS: Picnic table, fire pit

ASSIGNMENT: First come, first served; reservations recommended

REGISTRATION: At camp host station if staffed; if not, camp host will come around to collect fee; reserve sites by phone at 707-672-6018 up to 1 year in advance

AMENITIES: Nonpotable water, vault toilets, river access, two sites with RV hookups. No power. Plans are underway for showers and drinking water.

PARKING: At individual site

FEE: $15, $30 group sites, $5 extra vehicle

ELEVATION: 300'

RESTRICTIONS:

PETS: Dogs on leash

FIRES: In established pits or rings only

ALCOHOL: No restrictions

OTHER: Reservations made up to 3 weeks in advance

campground. In the heart of summer, the campground and day-use area are popular with folks looking for some cool river relief from soaring temperatures. Fishing for steelhead and salmon is popular, and a rafting outfit in Willow Creek offers numerous whitewater day-trip expeditions and multiday campout trips in the area, along the Trinity and Klamath Rivers (contact Bigfoot Rafting Company at 530-629-2263 or bigfootrafting.com).

The Trinity—a wide, fast-moving river flowing north toward the Klamath River—is a majestic sight. The campground's namesake, Tish Tang Creek, spills into it from the east, on the north side of the beach. When we camped here in June, the water was still quite cold, and signs warned of the dangerously swift currents—swimming is not advised until July, when the water slows down and warms up. The beach area is very rocky, so if you want to lounge about, the most comfortable option is a chair rather than a blanket. There aren't a lot of terrestrial activities in the immediate area; again, it's all about the river.

In this natural setting, you don't have to work to experience nature—it's all around, and all you need to do is become aware of it. Small lizards rule the campground, and you'll hear them scuttling about in the bushes. Birds are common, both in the campground and around the river, where we watched an osprey silently drop to the water and catch a fish, all in one graceful motion. California sister and swallowtail butterflies floated in the afternoon sunshine. Lucky campers may see bald eagles, otters, and beavers.

Willow Creek is a convenient last stop for campers headed to Tish Tang, offering basic camping amenities, including gas, groceries, and a few restaurants.

As you drive to Tish Tang from the coast, you seem to be heading deep into the mountains, but the climbing and descending mostly cancel each other out, and in the end you gain only about 300 feet in elevation. It gets good and hot at Tish Tang, so if you want cooler summer temperatures, you'll have to drive higher into the Shasta-Trinity National Forest.

The campground has undergone a good bit of change in the past few years. In 2017, tribal member Inker McCovey took over management of the campground and has since made significant headway in cleaning up, maintaining, and grooming it. Plans are under way for running water, showers, and even a camp store for the 2018 season and beyond. McCovey even goes out of his way to greet every guest in his native language. Still, it's a campground for those who don't mind a more rustic experience and are open to a wide range of guests (it isn't uncommon to find buff sunbathers down by the river). If you do decide to give Tish Tang a visit, chances are you will leave refreshed and revived from the healing qualities of the Trinity.

Tish Tang Campground

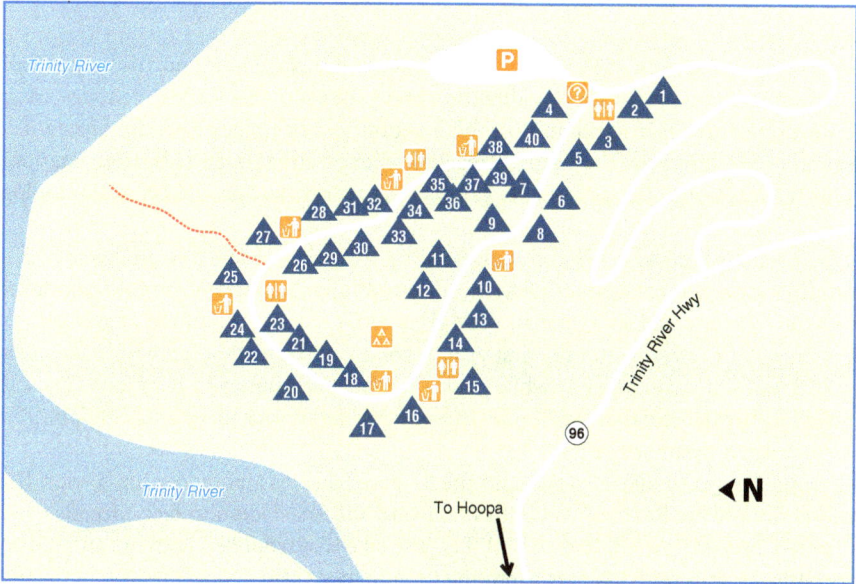

GETTING THERE

From Arcata on US 101 in Humboldt County, turn east onto CA 299. Drive east 40 miles to the town of Willow Creek, then turn left onto CA 96, signed to Hoopa. Drive north 8 miles, then turn right at the Tish Tang Campground sign. Continue downhill a short distance on the twisty road, to a fork in the road. Proceed to the left, into the campground.

GPS COORDINATES: N41° 01.052' W123° 30.148'

18

Castle Lake and Gumboot Campgrounds

Beauty ★★★★★ / Privacy ★★★★ / Spaciousness ★★★★ / Quiet ★★★★★ / Security ★★★ / Cleanliness ★★★

You've come to one of the most rugged and beautiful areas in California.

The towering white peak of Mount Shasta stands center stage in far north-central California, gathering attention from every direction and vantage point. And while there are great outdoor opportunities around and on this magnificent sleeping giant, the Shasta-Trinity Forest off its western shoulder holds a treasury of lakes, streams, and glacial formations.

One such treasure is Castle Lake. Famous the world over as UC Davis' Limnological Research Center, it resembles the high alpine lakes of the Swiss and Austrian Alps.

I first visited here as a kid and was awed by this lake, which was unlike any I'd seen before. The water is crystal clear due to the low levels of plant nutrients in the rocky lakebed. Across the pine-covered shoreline and cut-glass surface rises a mountain of granite against a clear blue sky. For years after my first visit, I wondered where that incredible lake resided; happily, I found it again one day while exploring the roads outside Mt. Shasta City. Often, a return visit to an area as an adult doesn't live up to memories made as a child, but Castle Lake once again mesmerized me.

Though I've yet to take a kayak onto the 47-acre lake, it's among my top to-dos. Seeing rafters and kayakers heading straight out toward the sheer granite face provides a great perspective on just how tall that rock cliff is. The lake is surrounded with firs and pines and offers lakeside trails until it smacks into the granite mountain.

Views of 14,180-foot Mount Shasta dominate the north-central California landscape.

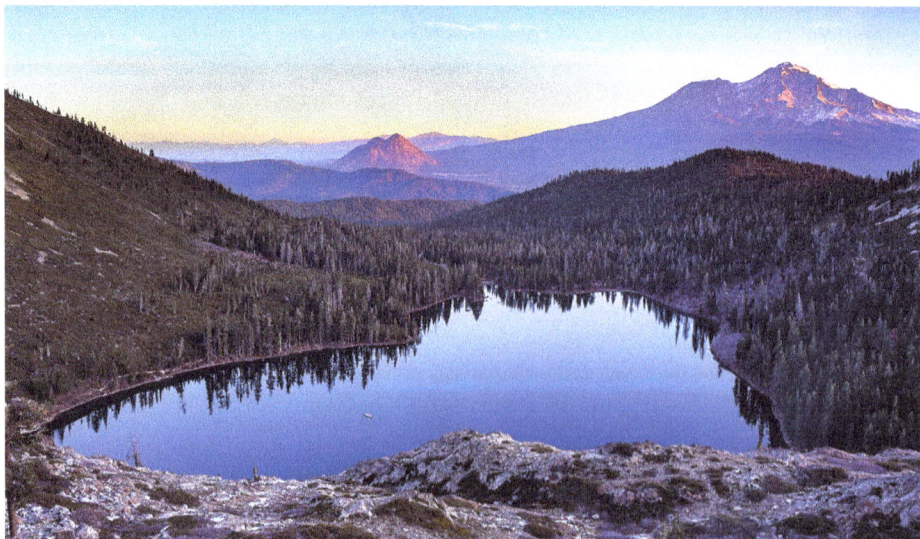

photographed by Vicki Mar Photography

KEY INFORMATION

LOCATION: West of Lake Siskiyou, Mt. Shasta, CA 96067

OPERATED BY: Shasta-Trinity National Forest, Shasta McCloud Management Unit

CONTACT: 530-926-4511; www.fs.usda.gov/stnf

OPEN: May–October (weather permitting)

SITES: Castle Lake: 6 sites for tents and RVs; Gumboot Lake: 8 sites, 4 for tents and RVs, 4 walk-in sites across creek

EACH SITE HAS: Picnic table, fire rings at Castle Lake only

ASSIGNMENT: First come, first served; no reservations

REGISTRATION: None

AMENITIES: Vault toilets, some wheelchair accessibility

PARKING: At individual site; parking lot for walk-in sites

FEE: None

ELEVATION: Castle Lake: 5,280'; Gumboot: 6,080'

RESTRICTIONS:

PETS: On leash

FIRES: With permit in fire ring

ALCOHOL: No restrictions

VEHICLES: RVs up to 16 feet

OTHER: No motors on lake; garbage must be packed out; no drinking water; 3-night stay limit at Castle Lake

---

Beneath the surface and against the cirque face, the lake drops 110 feet deep, dug out by the formative glaciers of ancient days. At the parking area, the water is less austere at only 10–15 feet—you can imagine with such a sharp underwater descent why there's such fascination about exploring the lake within the park's confines.

There's no camping on the lake, but sites are available less than a mile back down the mountain, keeping you close enough for frequent jaunts to the crystal waters, and hiking trails abound throughout the region.

Winter brings visitors to Castle Lake for snowshoeing, cross-country skiing, and ice-skating, and anglers arrive for some of the best ice fishing around. If you listen carefully, you might catch why a hollow moaning sound led American Indians to believe that an evil presence inhabited the lake. Today the sound is known to be the ice shifting and the wind roaming the rocky crevasses above the lake.

The Castle Lake area is also known for its vibrant display of red columbine, fawn lily, and Shasta penstemon in late spring to early summer. Trails lead into Castle Crags Wilderness Area and on to Castle Crags State Park.

Found on the south slope of Mount Eddy, not far along the same ridge of mountains but by way of a longer route by road, is the small but lovely Gumboot Lake. Another alpine treasure, this 7-acre lake offers some wonderful primitive campsites, without picnic tables or official fire rings, along the water or within view. This undeveloped camping area is a haven for nature lovers, with a wide variety of plants, birds, insects, and frogs. Take the informal trail and you might find blue heron near the lake or even bald eagles among the pines and firs.

Throw your line in either Gumboot or Castle Lake and the only fish you'll have a shot of pulling out is wild trout. Neither lake has been stocked since 2009 due to environmental concerns about the foothills yellow-legged frog. If good fishing is what you're after, take the Pacific Crest Trail 2.5 miles south to the Seven Lakes Basin. The Gumboot trailhead is right at camp.

W. A. Barr Road connects Castle and Gumboot Lakes and passes the larger, more developed, and more populated Lake Siskiyou. This is a nice stop for the day if you're in the mood for a refresher on civilization. Motorboats are allowed here, and boat rentals are available, as are camping, group sites, fishing, and beaches where you can enjoy the warm afternoons.

Visit Mt. Shasta City for shopping, mountain gear, crafts, and artwork. The restaurants are diverse, from the Black Bear Diner (offering the best in home-style cooking) to a number of ethnic restaurants and natural-food cafés.

However, I highly recommend that you spend the majority of your time as a true explorer of the high country. You've come to one of the most rugged and beautiful areas in California, so explore the roads, trails, and other alpine lakes while staying at or near Gumboot and Castle Lakes.

Castle Lake and Gumboot Campgrounds

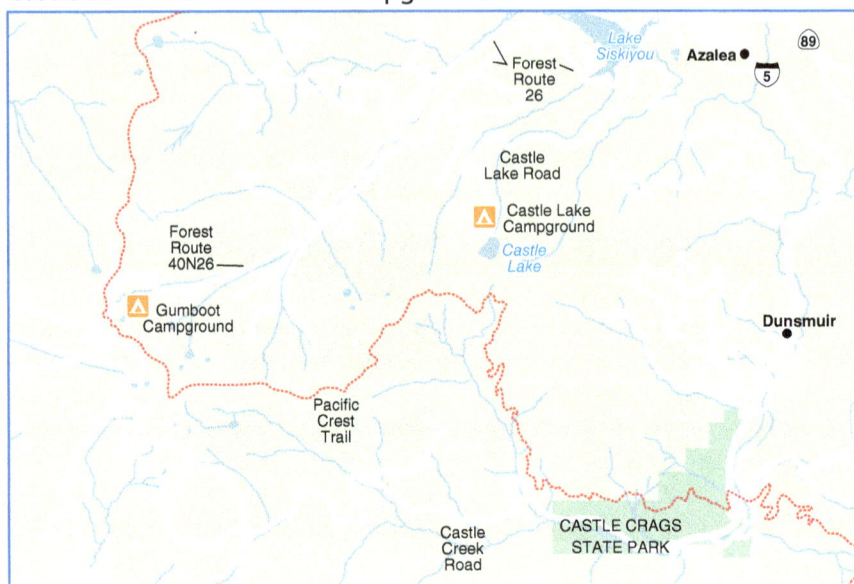

GETTING THERE

For Gumboot Lake: From Redding, head north 60 miles on I-5. Take Exit 738 and turn west across the overpass, then south on Old Stage Road, and bear right onto W. A. Barr Road, which becomes Forest Road 40N26. Drive 13 miles. Turn left at the fork in the road, and proceed the last 0.5 mile to the campground.

For Castle Lake: Follow directions above to W. A. Barr Road. Cross Box Canyon Dam, and then turn left on what starts as Ney Springs Road and becomes Castle Lake Road. Continue about 7 miles to the campground on the left.

GPS COORDINATES: CASTLE LAKE: N41° 14.108' W122° 22.802'
GUMBOOT LAKE: N41° 12.764' W122° 30.560'

19

Dillon Creek Campground

Beauty ★★★★★ / Privacy ★★★★ / Spaciousness ★★★ / Quiet ★★★ / Security ★★★★★ /
Cleanliness ★★★★

*Good steelhead fishing and a great swimming hole, right in the middle of the best
river rafting*

All rangers will tell you Dillon Creek Campground is a good campground. "Ah, Dillon," they say, smiling. "The river down there is nice." Rangers love Dillon because it is a model campground. The host's trailer sits right at the entrance to where the campsites file back along the hill. And, located by CA 96, Dillon is easy to patrol. I spoke to the campground host, who said, "We had an unruly bear here once, and I called for help on my mobile phone. The law was here in 10 minutes." Did they arrest the bear? I forgot to ask.

A steep trail leads down to Dillon Creek, where there is one great swimming hole near the campground, as well as dozens of more secluded ones upstream. Although Dillon Creek can flow ferociously in the spring flood, the current does not present the danger of the mighty Klamath that flows right across CA 89 from Dillon, where everybody goes for salmon and the famous steelhead.

Beginning in the fall, the name of the game here is steelhead. For anglers, this means the Klamath River in the winter, cold nights around a smoky campfire telling fish stories, and that one hard bite on the line that can only mean steelhead. What's a steelhead?

Summertime means swimming time at some of Northern California's best spots, on beautiful Dillon Creek.

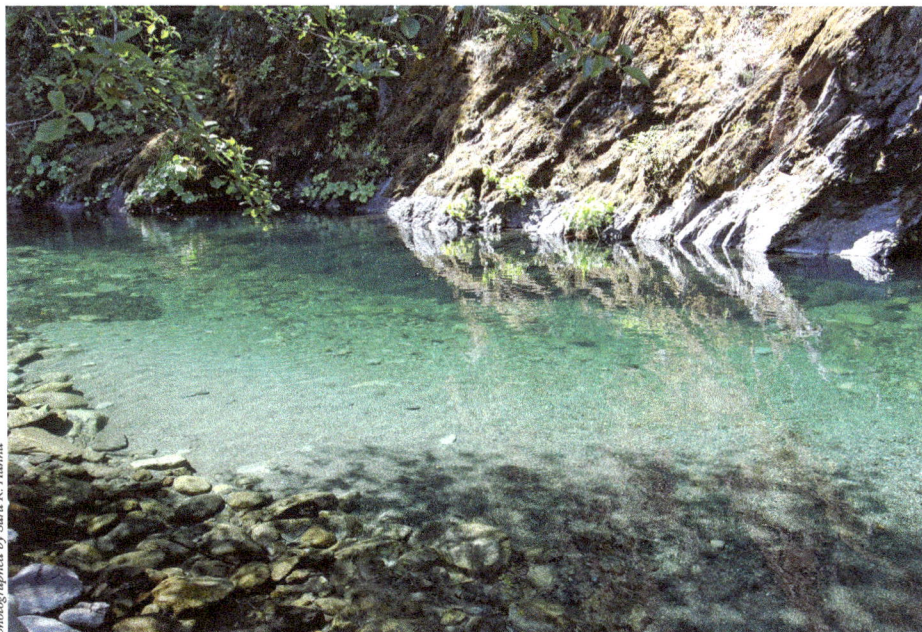

photographed by Sara K. Hanna

KEY INFORMATION

LOCATION: Approximately 76345 CA 96, Somes Bar, CA 95568

OPERATED BY: Six Rivers National Forest, Orleans Ranger District

CONTACT: 530-627-3291; www.fs.usda.gov/srnf

OPEN: May–October

SITES: 21 total: 11 sites for tents only and 10 sites for tents or RVs

EACH SITE HAS: Picnic table, fireplace, grills

ASSIGNMENT: Reserve at least 3 days in advance at recreation.gov; some may be available first come, first served

REGISTRATION: By entrance; reserve at 877-444-6777 or recreation.gov

AMENITIES: Water, vault toilets, wheelchair accessibility

PARKING: At individual site

FEE: $10 plus $5 day-use fee, $5 extra vehicle

ELEVATION: 1,780'

RESTRICTIONS:

PETS: On leash only

FIRES: In fireplace

ALCOHOL: No restrictions

VEHICLES: No trailers over 25 feet, no hookups

Steelhead are a kind of rainbow trout. Like salmon, steelhead spend some of their lives in the ocean, feeding and growing faster than their exclusively freshwater cousins, rainbow trout, then head up rivers like the Klamath to spawn. Steelhead average 10 pounds (some grow to 20 or more). Unlike salmon, steelhead do not die after spawning. They can come back two or three times to spawn again.

Steelhead and salmon look mostly alike. Steelhead have 9–12 bones or rays in their anal fin, and salmon have 13–19. (The anal fin is the bottom fin in front of the tail and behind the vent.) Steelhead have small, round, black spots on their back, and salmon have larger, irregular spots and lack the broad red stripe the steelhead get after being in freshwater for a while.

Peak months for catching big steelhead are January, February, and March. But littler ones (half-pounders) come into the Klamath in the spring and spend the summer in big river pools before spawning in the fall rains. Other little guys and some big mothers will come into the Klamath as early as August. How you fish steelhead depends on how the run is—and how your luck is. Once you hook a steelhead, it takes skill to land one, for steelhead are acrobatic, hard-fighting fish. Good luck! Of course, to improve the odds, ask around in Happy Camp (don't you just love the name of that town?) for a good fishing guide.

Last time I was in Dillon, the fall run of steelhead had not arrived. The campground host told me anglers were catching steelhead down near Somes Bar. Only mildly disappointed, we put on our water shoes and went down to the swimming hole. It was nice and hot. We had good fun working our way up Dillon Creek River, checking things out. We took a picnic, found a nice warm rock next to a clear pool, and hung out for the afternoon.

The next day, we found a trail that ran up the north side of Dillon Creek and followed it up a mile or so. Later I heard that this trail is used by the Fish and Game people, who hike up to where Dillon Creek forks to do a fish count. South of the campground entrance, Forest Service Road 13N35 heads up the shoulder of Dillon Mountain (4,679'). We hiked it until it got too steep and the sun got too hot.

There is also a trail that heads up the mountain behind the campground, but I couldn't find anyone who knew where it went. Basically, by the time you get as far out in the woods as Dillon Creek Campground, folks don't spend much time marking trails. And, since this is rugged-individualist country—land of tacked-together shacks tied to the Klamath River bank with rusty cables, and pot plantations among the redwoods—it is not a healthy idea to lunge blindly off into the woods. You might end up as fertilizer. Try to stick to the riverbank and to semiofficial trails or roads.

For adventure, try river rafting. Happy Camp is full of experienced outfits happy to take you down the river. I recommend going with one of them your first couple of times out before trying anything hasty. Proper equipment is a must; a helmet and life jacket can make a huge difference when you, your spouse, or your kid is dumped suddenly into the rapids.

Happy Camp has a good supermarket (as well as good hamburgers at the Western-style bar/café in town). I saw flyers up in town for folks who will take you gold panning and horseback riding. The Happy Camp Ranger Station has all the details. This little town seems friendly as well as happy.

Dillon Creek Campground

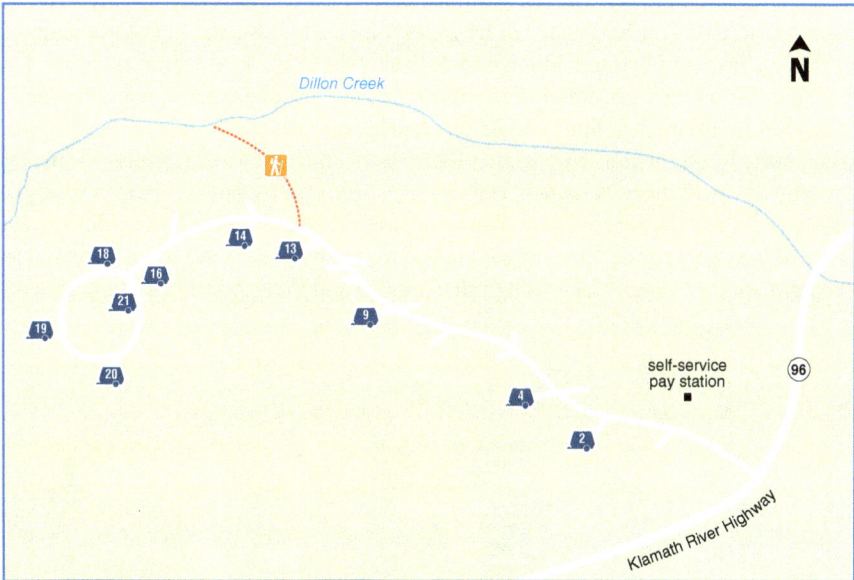

GETTING THERE

From Somes Bar, drive 15 miles north on CA 96. Or drive 22 miles south of Happy Camp on CA 96.

GPS COORDINATES: N41° 34.402' W123° 32.632'

20

Tree of Heaven Campground

Beauty ★★★★★ / Privacy ★★★★ / Spaciousness ★★★★★ / Quiet ★★★★★ / Security ★★★★★ / Cleanliness ★★★★★

Good for lawn sports, river rafting, fishing, and touring at nearby Yreka

The Tree of Heaven Campground comes as a stunning surprise. One moment you are driving along the Klamath in high sage country. You pass the relatively new Ash Creek Bridge (replaced in 2012 after 100 years), sweep around a curve, and see the U.S. Forest Service sign to the Tree of Heaven Campground. The entry drive drops suddenly down to the river, you reach the Tree of Heaven Campground, and suddenly you feel like you've been invited to an English garden party. All over there's green, tended grass. The campsites are on grass. There's room for baseball, and in the day-use area you'll find horseshoes, an open-pit barbecue, and a volleyball court with a net in tournament shape. Everything is neat and pruned. The wood-for-sale pile by the host trailer is squared away. The campers look well groomed. Even the campers' lap dogs are well maintained and strut around on their leads like little British marines.

The Klamath rolls by the campground like a watery muscle. Most campers swim right in front of the camp off the boat launch. Here the river runs pretty slowly, but everybody keeps a close eye on any kids, pets, or poor swimmers because this water is headed for the Pacific Ocean. Fishing can be great. One ranger I talked to said he was catching fish right and left in late September. Last time I was through there, I was told the fish were running but nobody

Ailanthus altissima, aka Tree of Heaven, is native to northeast and central China. Chinese immigrants living on the banks of the Klamath River in the 1800s imported and planted it along the banks at this beautiful campground. Leaves turn brilliant shades of red and yellow in autumn.

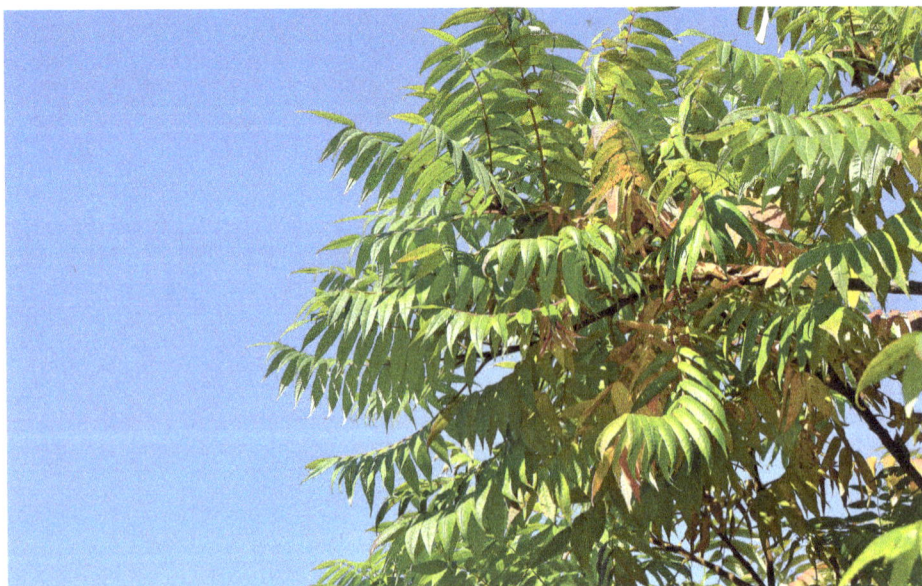

KEY INFORMATION

LOCATION: Klamath River Highway, 5 miles west of I-5, Yreka, CA 96097

OPERATED BY: Klamath National Forest, Happy Camp/Oak Knoll Ranger District

CONTACT: 530-493-2243; www.fs.usda.gov/klamath

OPEN: May–October

SITES: 21 total: 1 wheelchair-accessible site, 1 group site (nonreservable)

EACH SITE HAS: Picnic table, fireplace

ASSIGNMENT: First come, first served; reservations available (and recommended)

REGISTRATION: By entrance; reserve at 877-444-6777 or recreation.gov

AMENITIES: Water, vault toilets, boat ramp

PARKING: At individual site

FEE: $15

ELEVATION: 2,100'

RESTRICTIONS:

PETS: On leash only

FIRES: In fireplace

ALCOHOL: No restrictions

VEHICLES: Small RVs only; 2 vehicles/site, trailers included

OTHER: All food must be properly stored in approved containers; check weather conditions and water availability; no off-highway vehicle use; no livestock allowed; 14-day stay limit

was catching anything yet. A lady ranger said the salmon were pretty beat up by the time they get that far, but her kids always catch good-tasting steelhead trout.

There are hikes around Tree of Heaven, including an interpretive hike near the day-use area. Take the Tree of Heaven Trail that heads down by the river about 2 miles. It takes you to a good fishing place. But to really step out, you need to get in your car and head back toward I-5. Turn right on Ash Creek Bridge, which you passed on the way in. A mostly dirt road runs west down the south side of the Klamath. This is good hiking (as long as your dogs last) and great mountain biking. The road winds around with the river until it hits Walker Bridge about 18 miles downstream. On the way, you'll pass Humbug Creek Road, which is worth a look—assuming you're on your mountain bike and don't mind a climb, of course. By Walker Bridge on CA 96 is the Oak Knoll Ranger Station, so you can use the phone, beg for help, try to hitch a ride, or steel yourself for the climb back up to Tree of Heaven Campground.

The name of the game here is rafting. It's best to phone the Ranger Station a week or so in advance to get the name of a reputable outfitter and arrange a trip. Locals, of course, know the waters and use their own rafts. I firmly believe that discretion for strangers in these parts is the better part of valor. Spending a little money up front can save you a lot of grief later—especially if you bring your family along. The outfitters have helmets and life vests. Get it right the first time, and then maybe come back the next year with your own stuff.

Yreka (pronounce the Y, then say "reka," or be roundly mocked by the locals) is a major draw only 15 minutes away. The trick is not to get on I-5 when going to and from it. Not only is the exit confusing, but you lose all sense of "being" in Yreka or in Tree of Heaven. Yreka is a wonderful little town that was founded back in 1851 by Abraham Thompson, who watched in amazement as his grazing mules brought up flecks of gold tangled in the roots of the grass. In six weeks, 2,000 miners arrived, and soon there were 27 saloons in town (first things first!). Now there's a good sports bar on the corner of Miner and Main Streets.

In the Siskiyou County Museum, Yreka has the best small-museum exhibition of American Indian life and crafts I've ever seen. Then there are the eye-popping nuggets in the courthouse, all the incredible Victorian houses (walk, don't drive), and all of the very friendly people.

The tree that gives the campground its name is a Chinese tree (*Ailanthus altissima*) commonly called the Tree of Heaven. Chinese laborers planted them by gold mines and along railroad tracks. Known as a weed tree because it spreads by root suckers and "airplane propeller" seeds, the Tree of Heaven is attractive and indestructible.

Tree of Heaven Campground

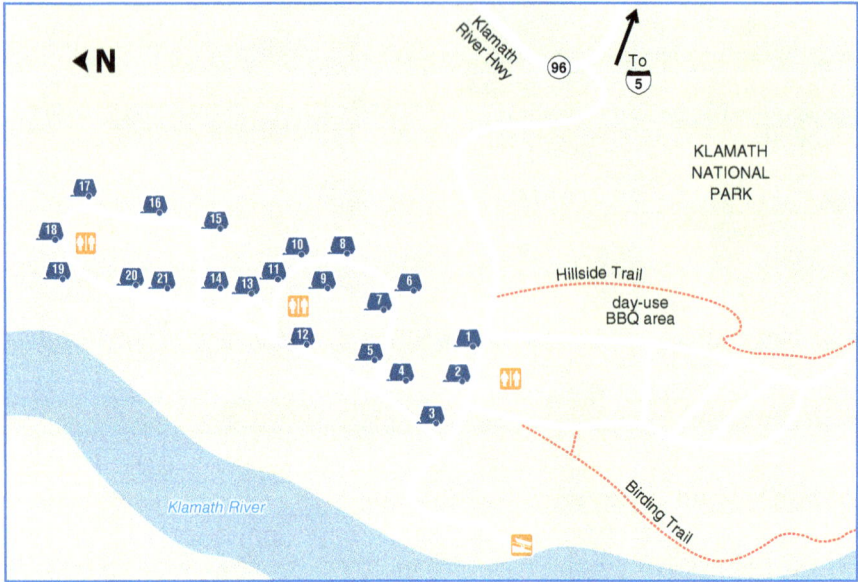

GETTING THERE

From Yreka, drive about 8 miles north on CA 263. Turn left (west) onto CA 96. Look for the Tree of Heaven Campground sign in 4.3 miles on the left. Be careful on the turn. Or take I-5 to Exit 786; head west (left) on Anderson Grade Road, and in 0.2 mile, turn left onto CA 96. In 6.5 miles, turn left into the campground.

GPS COORDINATES: N41° 49.925' W122° 39.568'

THE CASCADE RANGE

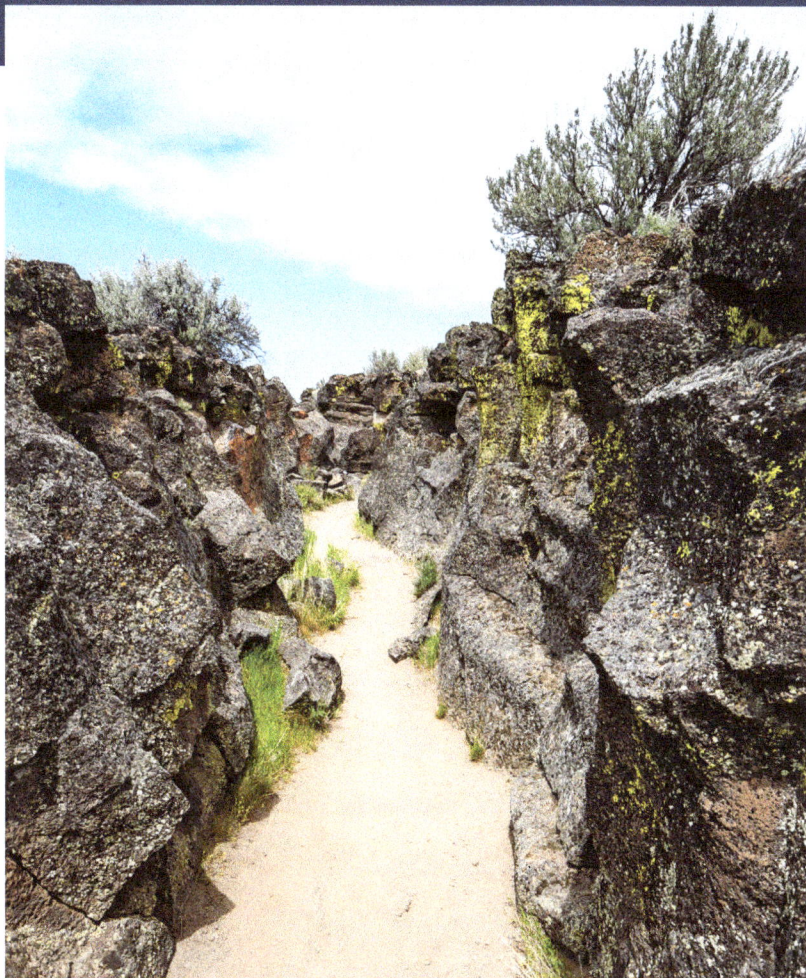

Hike through history and a natural lava fortress on Captain Jack's Stronghold trail in Indian Well National Monument *(see page 107)*.

21

Warner Valley Campground

Beauty ★★★★★ / Privacy ★★★★★ / Spaciousness ★★★★★ / Quiet ★★★★ / Security ★★★★★ / Cleanliness ★★★★

Read the camp register and become a believer—this campground is a jewel to cherish.

Warner Valley Campground is a great place to visit. It caters to tent campers (the road in is not recommended for trailers), and the bear boxes have helped decrease the number of bears. There is a ranger station a mile back down the road and a resort (Drakesbad Guest Ranch) a few hundred yards up the road. The trails are spectacular. Hot Springs Creek gurgles by the campground, lulling the tent camper to sleep, and the swimming is great. The sites are shaded but opened up, so you can get a sense of the land. Sites 1–6 are prime real estate by the creek, but the rest, on the other side of the road, offer privacy. The drinking water is cold and clean. Chester, with all the supplies a body could ever require, is a hop, skip, and a jump down the bucolic country road past little farms, old orchards, and rough little vacation homes. Good hikes splay out from the campground to just about everywhere. Or you can get in your car and explore Lassen Volcanic National Park, the most underused national park in the West.

Read the Warner Valley Campground register to see how revered it is: "Always come here, always will." "Dave's twentieth summer here." "Beautiful place to make a baby." "Trails are the best." "Lovely, quiet, serene." "Great swimming in Hot Springs Creek." "God's country." "Perfecto mundo." "Absolutely divine!" "Don't tell anyone about this place."

Hike up to Terminal Geyser, one of the closest geothermal features to Warner Valley Campground, and also one of the noisiest in Lassen Volcanic National Park.

KEY INFORMATION

LOCATION: Chester Warner Valley Road, 17 miles north of Chester in Mineral, CA 96063

OPERATED BY: Lassen Volcanic National Park

CONTACT: 530-595-4480; nps.gov/lavo

OPEN: Late May–October (weather permitting)

SITES: 17 sites for tents or small RVs

EACH SITE HAS: Picnic table, fire ring, food locker

ASSIGNMENT: First come, first served; no reservations

REGISTRATION: At entrance

AMENITIES: Water available mid-June–late September, vault toilets

PARKING: At individual site

FEE: $16 ($12 from early October to snow closure)

ELEVATION: 5,650'

RESTRICTIONS:

PETS: On leash only

FIRES: In fire ring

ALCOHOL: No restrictions

VEHICLES: Not recommended for trailers or RVs

OTHER: Don't leave food out; use food lockers

One minor disappointment is the fishing; it's not great in Lassen Volcanic National Park. Since the mid-1970s the Park Service has not stocked most of the park's lakes and streams. However, near Warner Valley Campground, just outside the park, is some fine fishing. Try the Caribou Wilderness to the east—hike in to the lakes. Caribou, Echo, and Silver Lakes are well stocked, but folks can drive to them, so they get heavy play. To the south are Lake Almanor and Deer Creek, both of which have great fishing.

OK, so you can't live off the land at Warner Valley Campground. The only local food supply in the immediate area is the restaurant at the Drakesbad Guest Ranch. It provides breakfast, lunch, and dinner for hikers and campers; reservations are recommended, as space is limited.

Rooms at the ranch run about $175 per person per night for three meals, a room, and access to the geothermally heated pool. Horseback riding and massages are extra. Still, Drakesbad is legendary and should be on the agenda of a "do everything" California explorer at least once in a lifetime. The place (settled by a relative of both Sir Francis Drake and the more contemporary Jim Drake of Santa Monica, inventor of the Windsurfer) is more than a century old. People come here the same week in summer year after year. So reserve ahead in the summer. Call 866-999-0914 or visit drakesbad.com for more info.

A fun little hike from Warner Valley Campground is up to Boiling Springs Lake. The trailhead is on the left, a few hundred yards past the campground on the way to the visible Drakesbad Resort. Follow the obvious trail, and cross Hot Springs Creek on the bridge. Reach a junction. A right takes you to Drakesbad Lake, Dream Lake, and Devils Kitchen. Go left and reach another junction, where the trail to the right goes to Drake Lake and, again, Devils Kitchen (another must-do hike, with fumaroles and mud pots). Follow the signs, and you will soon smell and hear Boiling Springs Lake before you arrive. The rotten-egg smell is the hydrogen sulfide from sulfur in the rising gases. The "bumping" sound is from the mud pots, which open and close like some monstrous earthen eye. Here's a hell even an atheist can believe in. The water is hot and yellow and green (yellow from opal and iron oxide, and green from algae). It is hot enough to scald and kill you. Stay on the trail—you don't want to fall through the thin crust and land in an incipient mud pot.

The last time I was at Warner Valley Campground was in September, and we had the place to ourselves. I swam in the pool just below the wooden bridge crossing Hot Springs Creek at the beginning of the Boiling Springs Lake Trail. Other times, when the campground was busier, we went downstream and found great pools off the road below the ranger station.

Weather here can be dicey. Come prepared for both hot and cold, and phone ahead to make sure the campground is open, as the Lassen area is notorious for being snowed in through early summer.

Warner Valley Campground

GETTING THERE

From Chester on CA 36, just east of the Feather River, head west on Feather River Drive by the fire station. After 0.6 mile veer left onto Chester Warner Valley Road, and then in 5.5 miles bear right at the next junction to stay on Warner Valley Road. Continue another 9.9 miles into the park and to Warner Valley Campground. (You will pass Warner Valley Ranger Station on the way.)

GPS COORDINATES: N40° 26.527′ W121° 23.615′

22

Juniper Lake Campground

Beauty ★★★★★ / Privacy ★★★★ / Spaciousness ★★★★★ / Quiet ★★★★★ / Security ★★★★★ / Cleanliness ★★★★★

It's the most pristine campground in Lassen Volcanic National Park, but it's the hardest to get to, so come prepared.

Come to Lassen Volcanic National Park and camp at Juniper Lake Campground because it offers the least-crowded camping, hiking, and fishing in the park. Juniper Lake, blue and deep, is by Lassen Peak, Mount Harkness, and Saddle Mountain. Until recently, in geologic time, Juniper Lake was not even a lake. About 200,000 years ago, all that was here was a depression with hundreds of feet of ice cap and icy fingers heading down into Warner Valley. The area warmed up, and a stream ran through the basin. Nearby volcanic Mount Harkness hadn't erupted, but when it did, it dammed up the south part of the basin, and voilà! Juniper Lake was born.

The last 8 miles into the Juniper Lake Campground are not great driving, but if you go slowly you can make it in any kind of vehicle. You just have to take your time and be careful. Plan on taking an hour to make that last 8 miles. Once you scale down your expectations, rough road traveling becomes enjoyable. Suddenly you can see the trees and the birds instead of a rushing green blur. Let about 5 PSI of air out of each tire if you want to stop your dentures from rattling. And remember, a nasty road is what keeps Juniper Lake from being a tourist hot spot. This is deliberate. Years ago, Lassen Volcanic National Park decided not to stock its lakes and not to fix up its roads, hoping to stanch the stampede and keep the park as pristine as possible.

Do all your shopping in Chester before you drive into Juniper Lake, because you won't want to pop out for hot dog buns. Filtering water is lots of work as well—it takes a ton of pumping to filter out a quart of water.

It's worth the effort to get to Juniper Lake, where you can set up camp right on the water's edge.

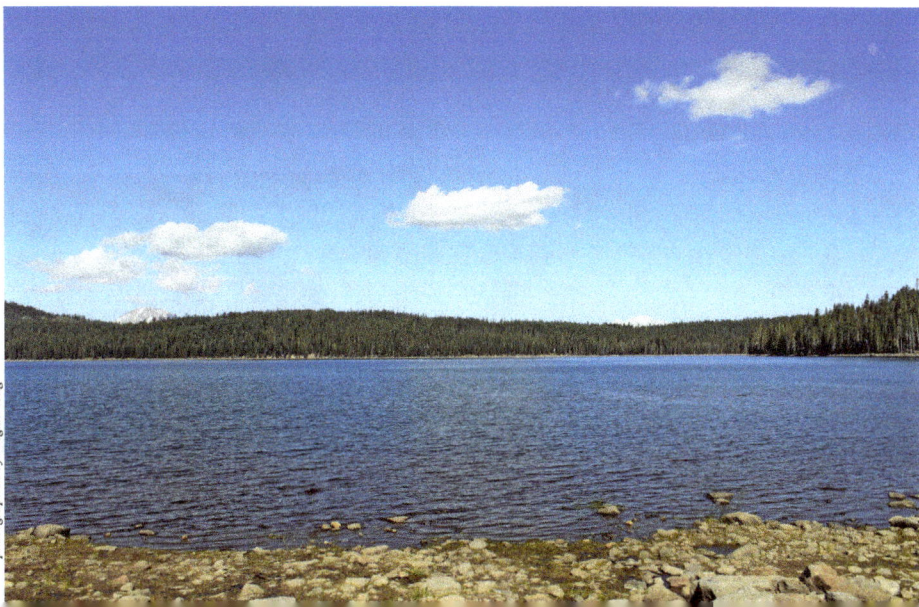

photographed by Megan Tong

KEY INFORMATION

LOCATION: Chester Juniper Lake Road, 12 miles north of Chester, CA 96020

OPERATED BY: Lassen Volcanic National Park

CONTACT: 530-595-4480; nps.gov/lavo

OPEN: July 1–mid-October (weather permitting)

SITES: 18 tent sites, 2 group sites

EACH SITE HAS: Picnic table, fire ring, food locker

ASSIGNMENT: Tent sites are first come, first served (no reservations); group sites must be reserved at least 4 days ahead

REGISTRATION: By entrance

AMENITIES: Vault toilets

PARKING: At individual site

FEE: $20 park entrance vehicle fee (good for 7 days), $12 camping fee

ELEVATION: 6,792'

RESTRICTIONS:

PETS: On leash only; no pets on trails, on beach, or in water

FIRES: In fire ring

ALCOHOL: No restrictions

VEHICLES: Small campers only; no RVs

OTHER: Check weather; use food lockers or other approved containers; rough dirt road not recommended for trailers; no water—bring your own

Come prepared for any kind of weather. At any time, it can be either freezing or like August on the Riviera. Bring winter sleeping bags with a sheet—if it is hot, use the sheet over you and lie on the bag. If it's cold, crawl into the warm sleeping bag.

Be sure to hike up to Crystal Lake. This hike is only about 0.5 mile, but it's a killer. When you arrive, you'll need a swim regardless of the weather. Fortunately, Crystal Lake is warm. Why? I don't know. Juniper Lake is icy. Maybe Crystal Lake is warm because it is on a south-facing slope. Bring a lunch and stay all day. Some say Crystal Lake has trout—I didn't see anyone catch anything, but folks were fishing.

The hike up Mount Harkness is another steep climb (about 4 miles round-trip). Catch the trail right from the campground. Hike up through the firs and pines until the woods open up into slopes of gray-rock lava from Mount Harkness. Keep hiking up until you hit

Bring your kayak, canoe, or inflatable raft to Juniper Lake, where motorboats are prohibited, and enjoy beautiful paddling on glassy waters.

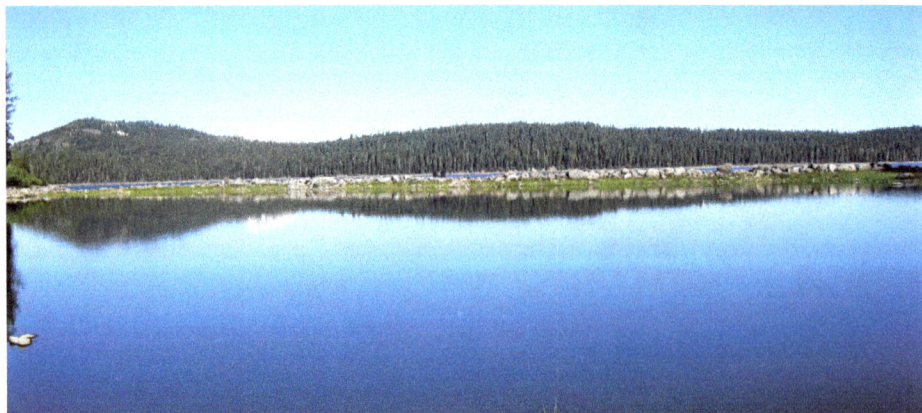

photographed by Russell Baldon

the cinder cone, and then head west, up through hemlocks to the ridge. From there it's up another 10 minutes to the fire lookout on the rim. From the lookout you can see just about the whole park. On the way back, a loop trail goes left and down to Juniper Lake. When you hit the lake, head east back to the campground. This loop is another mile or two longer than going back the way you came in.

Another good hike is around Juniper Lake, and this is more of a trek than one would expect. We underestimated the distance and forgot a lunch. The whole loop is about 6 miles, and there is enough up and down that we took 3 hard hours to complete the trail–cottage access road back to the campground. There is a rocky point on the Mount Harkness end of the lake, where we went swimming in the cold water. After involuntary gasps of shock came welcome numbness and then the exhilaration that keeps all those Nordic countries on their toes.

I heartily recommend bringing any rubber flotation device you can afford that will get your highly vulnerable body onto the gorgeous blue lake but out of the water. Think small inflatable boat. Never set your device down on sharp shale or pine needles—and come prepared with a repair kit.

Juniper Lake Campground

GETTING THERE

From Chester on CA 36, just east of the Feather River, head west on Feather River Drive by the fire station. After 0.6 mile veer right at the Y onto Juniper Lake Road and go 11 miles to Juniper Lake Campground on your left.

GPS COORDINATES: N40° 27.071' W121° 17.677'

23

Crater Lake Campground

Beauty ★★★★★ / Privacy ★★★★ / Spaciousness ★★★★ / Quiet ★★★★★ / Security ★★★★★ / Cleanliness ★★★★

In the fall, when the aspens go gold, this little campground is pretty and fun.

Crater Lake Campground has the most unexpected charm. You drive off CA 44 across a railroad track toward a mountain in the distance. The mostly dirt road (only 7 miles) winds up around a volcanic cone. Rough only in places, the road brings you to the lip of the cone in a short time, and you can look down on 27 acres of the prettiest little lake surrounded by aspens turning gold in the fall.

This is a small campground—only 17 campsites, and most of them are pitched wrong or too small for even small RVs, so this is prime tent camping. The sites are sprinkled up and down the loop to the lake's edge. The last time I was there, in September, we camped right on the lakeshore—no one else was there. The aspens (*Populus tremuloides*) were turning orange, yellow, and red against the black volcanic rock of the crater—beautiful.

California's Crater Lake is part of the great lava plateau, which includes Lassen Volcanic National Park and Lava Beds National Monument in Northern California and Crater Lake National Park (not our Crater Lake), in Oregon. Lassen Peak last erupted in May 1914 for a seven-year cycle of sporadic outbursts. When will it go off again? Soon, in geologic time, but nobody knows for certain.

Part of Crater Lake Campground's charm is being out in the middle of nowhere. The nearest reliable food supply is Susanville, an authentic cowboy town that manages to have a modern supermarket and a Bank of America. Gas, beer, and ice can be had at Old Station, off CA 44 at the junction of CA 89. But if you want fresh meat, only Susanville will do.

Stunning stands of aspen trees make this campground a must-visit in late September.

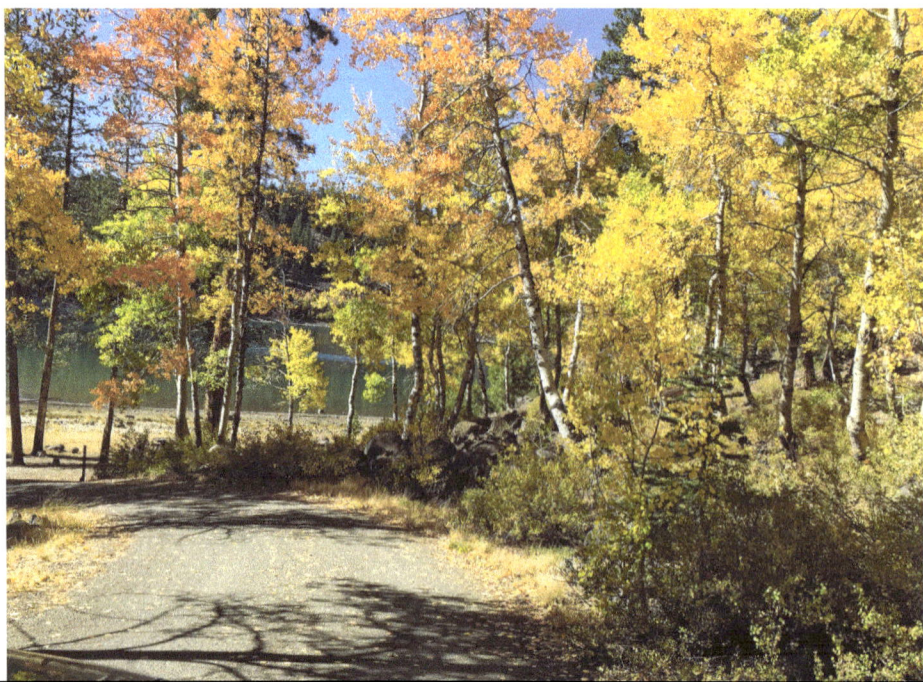

KEY INFORMATION

LOCATION: Forest Road 32N08, 6 miles north of CA 44, Susanville, CA 96130

OPERATED BY: Lassen National Forest, Eagle Lake Ranger District

CONTACT: 530-257-4188; www.fs.usda.gov/lassen

OPEN: June–October

SITES: 17 sites for tents or small campers

EACH SITE HAS: Picnic table, fireplace

ASSIGNMENT: First come, first served; no reservations accepted

REGISTRATION: By entrance

AMENITIES: Hand-pumped well water, vault toilets

PARKING: At individual site

FEE: $10

ELEVATION: 6,800'

RESTRICTIONS:

PETS: On leash only

FIRES: In fireplace

ALCOHOL: No restrictions

VEHICLES: No trailers over 20 feet; no gas motors on lake

Fishing on Crater Lake is pretty good, especially after it is stocked—and the 94-foot-deep lake hosts freshwater crawdads that in good years can be trapped for a one-crawdad, one-bite meal. A ranger I spoke to says their numbers go up and down—in the 1980s the crustaceans were especially prolific.

There is hiking around the lake. Back where the access road comes over the lip of the cone, there are several lumber roads heading out north. We walked all of them then tried some cross-country trekking and found it easy. You can easily hike through the patches of pine down into Harvey Valley or Pine Creek Valley. Still, I think of Crater Lake Campground as a one-night stop at an impossibly beautiful spot or a place to springboard by car to other adventures (like all of Lassen Volcanic National Park).

There is a beguiling island out in the middle of the lake. To get there, you'll need a watercraft. A canoe or kayak will do fine, as will an inflatable craft of some sort. You can have lots of fun floating around the tiny lake, fishing or reading, or sunbathing on the island, with an occasional dip into the freezing water. On a nice day there is nothing better than the hot sun on your body and the feeling of the cold water through a few inches of insulating soft air compressed by the not-too-thick sides of your blow-up raft or kayak (buy the inexpensive electric pump that runs off your car's cigarette lighter).

Good hiking, biking, and horseback riding are found nearby, on the Bizz Johnson Trail along the Susan River and the old Fernley & Lassen Railroad route from Susanville to Duck Lake, 4 miles north of Westwood. The Eagle Lake Ranger Station, at the intersection of CA 36 and Eagle Lake Road/County Road A1, can provide the Bizz Johnson Trail brochure, along with information on where to access the trail and rent bicycles or horses in Susanville.

Find more good hiking in Lassen Volcanic National Park at the Butte Lake trailheads, just a short way from Crater Lake Campground. Go out to CA 44, then head west a few miles to Forest Route 32N21. This road climbs 2.4 miles to Butte Creek Campground then 4.1 miles to Butte Lake Ranger Station.

An easy hike from the north side of the Butte Lake parking lot is the trail to Bathtub Lake (warm, safe swimming). Climb about 500 yards and you'll see two small lakes. The northernmost one is Bathtub, and both lakes will do for swimming. There are other trails from this area for more ambitious hikers (get information at the ranger station).

For another great expedition, take CA 44 and CA 36 east toward Susanville, then A1 north to Eagle Lake. Go right on Gallatin Road and find the beach and marina. A good boat with a motor costs about $70 per day, and you could spend a week fishing for the singular lake trout and exploring the miles of shore.

Crater Lake Campground

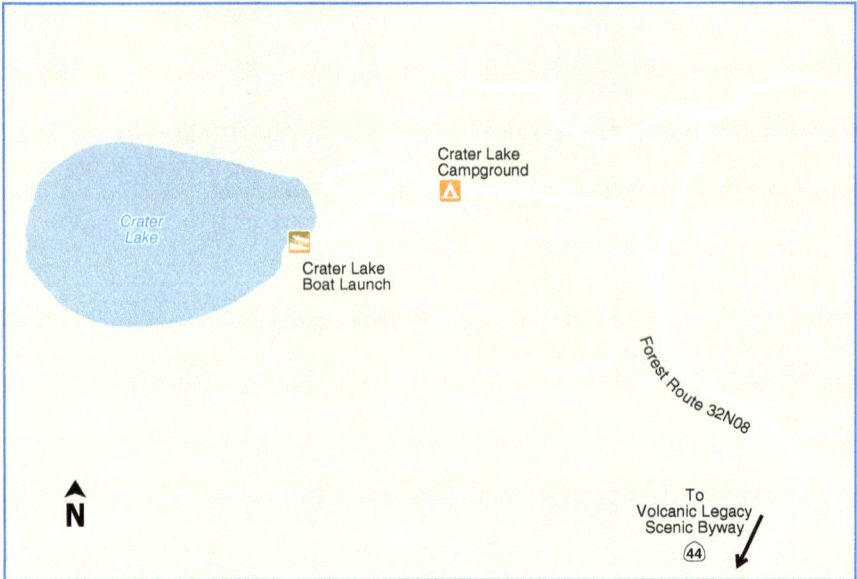

GETTING THERE

From Susanville, head 6 miles west on CA 36, then turn right to go another 22 miles west on CA 44 to the Bogard Work Center. Turn right on FR 32N08 and follow FR 32N08 north 7 miles to the Crater Lake Campground. Note: The roads here are rather rough, so take caution.

GPS COORDINATES: N40° 37.610' W121° 2.565'

24

Aspen Grove and Merrill Campgrounds

Beauty ★★★★★ / Privacy ★★★★★ / Spaciousness ★★★★★ / Quiet ★★★★ / Security ★★★★★ / Cleanliness ★★★★★

True destination campgrounds—you have to work to get there, and you'll want to stay for at least a week.

Eagle Lake is so uniquely beautiful that you have to go there, and it is so far from anywhere that you have to stay awhile. Don't bother lugging food supplies all the way to Eagle Lake—buy everything in nearby downtown Susanville, a town so Western that you'll expect Wyatt Earp to saunter out of one of the square brick buildings on Main Street in his bowler hat, toting a six-gun. Then you'll look around and see the supermarket, gas station, and bank. All the same, Susanville is a real cowboy town.

There are two ways into Eagle Lake from Susanville. One is up County Road A1 off CA 36, and the other is up Merrillville Road off CA 139. Both routes take you through a pass where you'll see Eagle Lake—the second-largest natural freshwater lake in California (Lake Tahoe is split by a state boundary). All the campgrounds are down on the south end of the lake—all connected by a great bicycle path that winds its way through the woods and lakeshore. What a beautiful place!

The campgrounds—Aspen Grove, Eagle, Merrill, and Christie—are run by the Lassen College Foundation to raise scholarship money and give Lassen Community College students

Spacious, flat sites at Merrill Campground (such as site 72, pictured here) provide little natural shade but can get you front-door access to beautiful Eagle Lake with excellent sunset views.

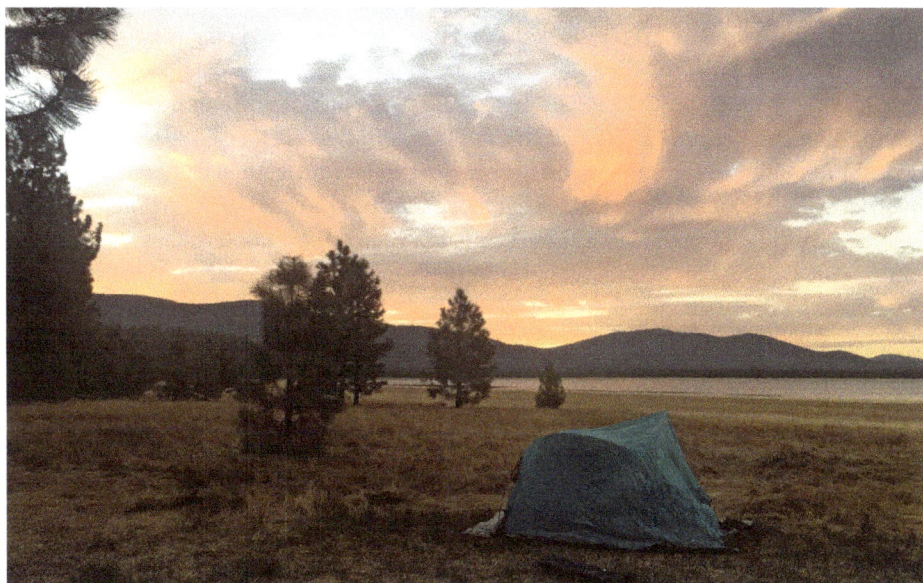

KEY INFORMATION

LOCATION: Eagle Lake Road, 13 miles north of CA 36, Susanville, CA 96130

OPERATED BY: Lassen National Forest, Eagle Lake Ranger District

CONTACT: Eagle Lake Ranger Station 530-257-4188; marina 530-825-3454; www.fs.usda.gov/lassen; eaglelakerecreationarea.com

OPEN: May–October (depending on road and weather conditions)

SITES: Aspen Grove: 27 sites; Merrill: 170 sites, 2 group sites

EACH SITE HAS: Picnic table, fire ring

ASSIGNMENT: Some sites take reservations; some are strictly walk-in

REGISTRATION: At entrance; reserve at 877-444-6777 or recreation.gov

AMENITIES: Water, flush toilets, wheelchair accessible, some full hookups (Merrill)

PARKING: Near individual site at Aspen, at individual site at Merrill

FEE: Aspen Grove $20; Merrill $20–$35; $8 nonrefundable reservation fee

ELEVATION: 5,100'

RESTRICTIONS:

PETS: On leash only (no pets on trails)

FIRES: In fireplace

ALCOHOL: No restrictions

VEHICLES: No RVs (tent only) at Aspen; no length limit at Merrill

---

hands-on recreation and parks management experience. It really shows. The whole camping experience at Eagle Lake feels clean, intelligent, and supremely enjoyable.

Aspen Grove Campground, for tent camping only, is a pretty little place on a knoll near the swimming beach and the marina. There's a store with showers, a laundromat, and bicycles to rent. Eagle Campground is nearby, maybe a quarter of a mile from the marina, but too near the road to suit me. The last time I was at the lake, we camped down at Merrill Campground, which is for RVs and tents together. Merrill became my family's favorite campground in California. Why? We liked scanning the skies for bald eagles and watching the osprey family ceaselessly swinging over the lake looking for fish. We liked our wide-open campsite, perfect for a pickup game of T-ball, and we loved being close to the water and the bike path.

Merrill is even better than Aspen Grove. For one thing, it's nice to be away from the marina. There is less boat and vehicle traffic. The campsites are all well spaced, and if you want more solitude, you can camp off the beach. If you want lakefront camping, remember to make a reservation. The sun and the light reflecting off the water can be a problem. There is some cover, but bring shade—a shade tent, a sombrero, or an umbrella that fits onto your beach chair. Don't forget to bring along buckets of sunscreen to slop on your exposed limbs.

Of course, many sites are first come, first served. You can also camp in a reservable site if you arrive and find it empty. Just check with the reservations host (in a separate trailer from the campground host), who will tell you if the site is open for the day. The best plan is to arrive, find a site that you would be happy with, park the car, and then nose around to see if you can find something better.

Next, get out your fishing rod. The fishing is reputedly great. Although I did not personally wash a worm—and did hear some anglers grousing—Eagle Lake has a reputation for the famous Eagle Lake rainbow trout. Apparently, the lake water is alkaline, which gives this subspecies of trout an extraordinary flavor.

Merrill Campground and Aspen Grove Campground

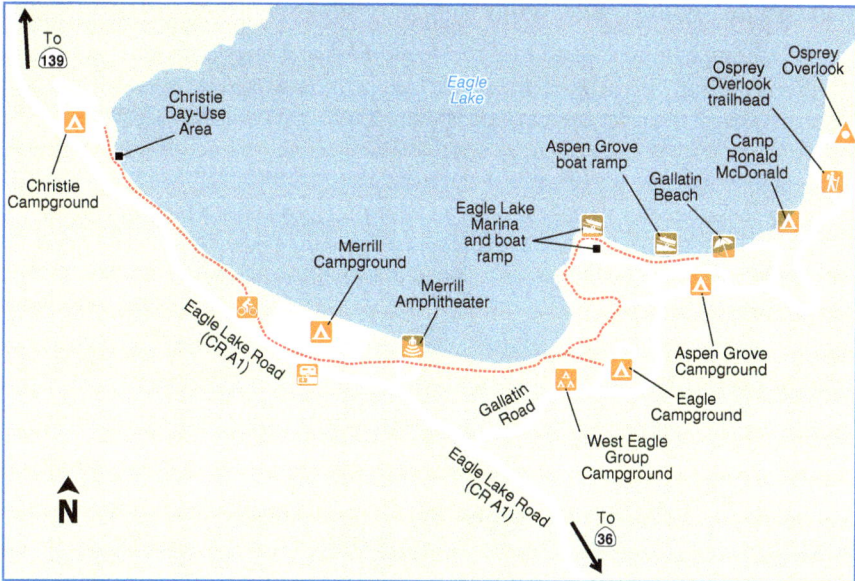

To (139)

Christie Campground

Christie Day-Use Area

Eagle Lake

Osprey Overlook trailhead

Osprey Overlook

Aspen Grove boat ramp

Camp Ronald McDonald

Gallatin Beach

Eagle Lake Marina and boat ramp

Merrill Campground

Merrill Amphitheater

Eagle Lake Road (CR A1)

Aspen Grove Campground

Eagle Campground

Gallatin Road

West Eagle Group Campground

Eagle Lake Road (CR A1)

To (36)

N

Aspen Grove Campground

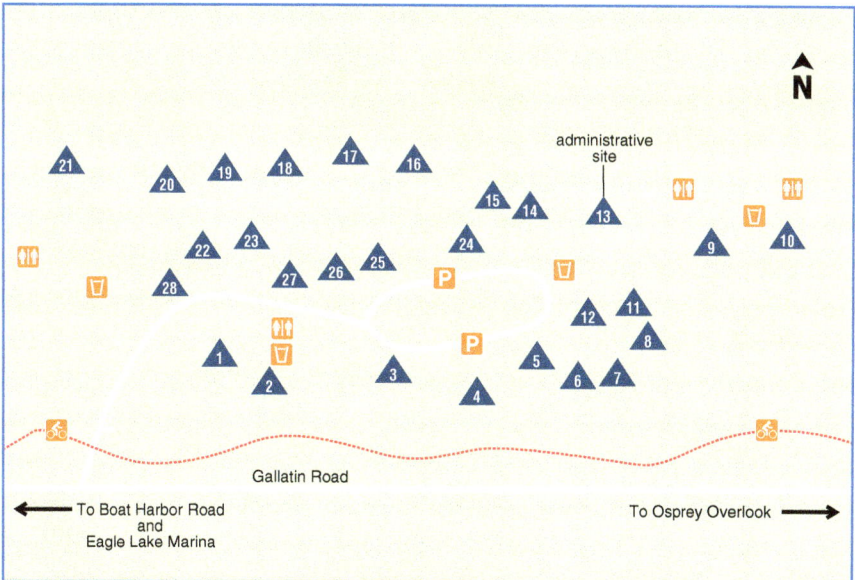

administrative site

21 20 19 18 17 16

15 14 13

22 23 24 9 10

28 27 26 25

P

1 2 3 4 5 6 7 8 11 12

Gallatin Road

To Boat Harbor Road and Eagle Lake Marina

To Osprey Overlook

N

The American Indians were always leery of Eagle Lake. Maybe it was the taste of the trout, or maybe it was the earthquake activity around Eagle Lake. In any case, they never established permanent camps here. The Maidu and Paiute would cruise through for a little fishing or hunting but didn't stay long. They believed that a huge Loch Ness–style serpent lived in the lake. They also believed that Eagle Lake was connected to faraway Pyramid Lake by an underground river. Pyramid Lake is about 100 miles away in Nevada. What gives this legend credence is that contemporary scientists can't seem to account for the apparently interdependent changing water levels in the two lakes.

To really get out and explore Eagle Lake in its entirety, you need a boat with a motor. The Eagle Lake Marina (530-825-3454) rents aluminum fishing boats for about $75/half day or $110/full day; the boats have to be returned an hour before the store closes. It's worth it to get out on this beautiful lake.

Merrill Campground

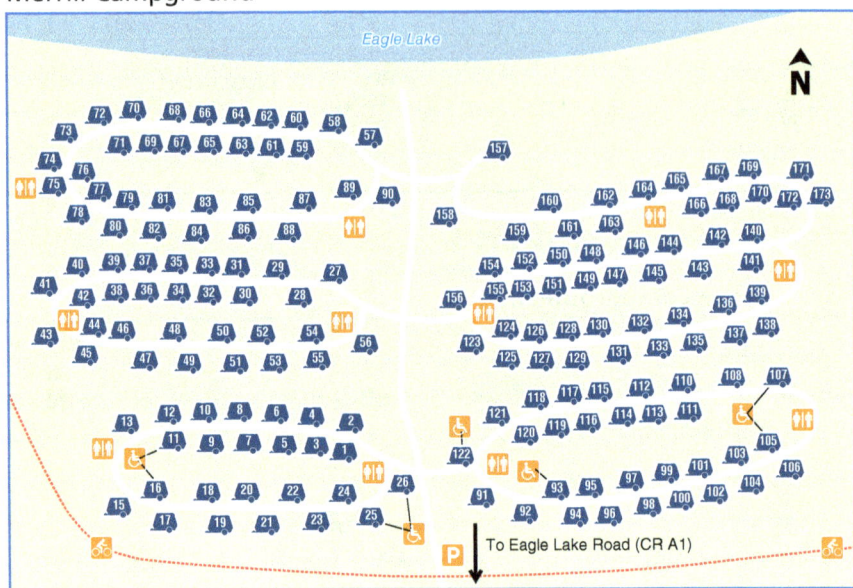

GETTING THERE

From Susanville, go 2.3 miles west on CA 36, then 13.3 miles north on County Road A1 (Eagle Lake Road) to Eagle Lake. To reach Merrill Campground, continue on Eagle Lake Road 1 mile or so. To reach Aspen, turn right on Gallatin Road and go 1.5 miles or so, past Eagle Campground.

GPS COORDINATES: ASPEN GROVE: N40° 33.323' W120° 46.437'
MERRILL: N40° 32.909' W120° 48.721'

25

McArthur–Burney Falls Memorial State Park Campgrounds

Beauty ★★★★★ / Privacy ★★★ / Spaciousness ★★★★★ / Quiet ★★★ / Security ★★★★★ / Cleanliness ★★★★

The queen of Northern California state campgrounds. Teddy Roosevelt called the nearby falls the "Eighth Wonder of the World."

Come to McArthur–Burney Falls Memorial State Park in the summer armed with reservations and children. You need reservations to get a campsite, and children to join all the other kids playing around the campsites, hiking the trails, and cavorting on the beautiful beach by the marina. However, in the fall or spring, McArthur–Burney Falls offers peace and quiet. It is a premium state park with good swimming, fishing, and hiking, as well as comfortable camping with hot showers.

Lake Britton is a reservoir, but it is uniquely fed (design courtesy of Ma Nature) by an underground spring that fills the reservoir and keeps the 129-foot Burney Falls flowing. Back east in the Finger Lakes (upstate New York) we have falls like Burney all over the place, but we don't have black swifts building rare inland nests of lichens on the cliffs. Nor do we have water ouzels (*Cinclus mexicanus*) diving into the creek to walk along the bottom while feeding. The birds hold their wings partially open, and the current pressing on their wings

Burney Falls, fed by subterranean springs, cascades 129 feet over plant-covered lava rock into a strikingly clear, blue pool. The falls are always flowing, always cold (42°F), and always spectacular.

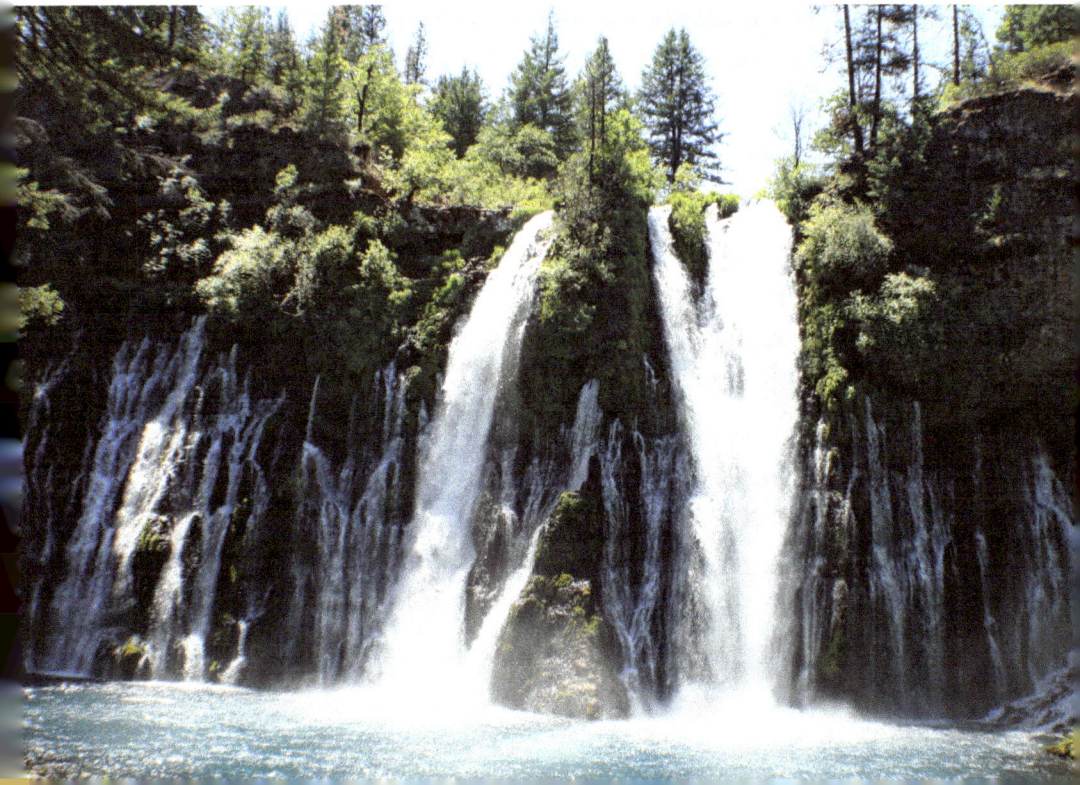

KEY INFORMATION

LOCATION: 24898 CA 89, Burney, CA 96013

OPERATED BY: McArthur–Burney Falls Memorial State Park

CONTACT: 530-335-2777; www.parks.ca.gov

OPEN: Year-round

SITES: 102 sites for tents or RVs up to 32 feet, 24 cabins with tent sites, 7 wheelchair-accessible sites

EACH SITE HAS: Picnic table, fireplace, food locker

ASSIGNMENT: First come, first served; reservations recommended

REGISTRATION: By entrance; reserve at 800-444-7275 or reservecalifornia.com

AMENITIES: Wi-Fi service near visitor center, water, flush toilets, coin-operated showers, firewood for sale, dump stations

PARKING: At individual site

FEE: $35, $30 off-season, $93.50 for site with small 2-person cabin, $115.50 for site with large 4-person cabin, $8 nonrefundable reservation fee, $8 extra vehicle

ELEVATION: 2,800'

RESTRICTIONS:

PETS: Dogs allowed on leash only

FIRES: In fireplace

ALCOHOL: No restrictions

VEHICLES: 2/site

OTHER: Reservations available mid-May–mid-September; first come, first served the rest of the year; 14-day stay limit

---

helps hold them down. They can go as deep as 20 feet and stay down for a minute before shooting up into the sky like a rocket.

On Lake Britton, which has good fishing (rent canoes, paddleboats, and motorboats at the park marina), look for great blue herons, Canada geese, and a multitude of ducks and grebes. Bald eagles visit in the winter, when the weather gets too rough for them up in Canada. In the campground, we saw redheaded woodpeckers, evening grosbeaks, and a host of other birds. At night we heard the great horned owl, a creature with a 5-foot wingspan capable of kidnapping a small dog. Yet the owl is constantly bullied by crows. How? Tough and clever, the crows attack together.

Around the campground you will find some good hikes—especially the popular Fall Creek Trail. This is a 1.2-mile self-guided interpretive loop that tours the creek canyon. Avoid this trail at all costs in the summer, except to access the trail that runs down the canyon to the beach on Lake Britton. At other times, this loop is astonishingly beautiful.

Another quick walk is up the Headwaters Trail to the underground spring and reservoir revered by the Ilmawi people living in nearby villages. The Ilmawi dug deep pits in deer trails to trap big game, so the first whites called the Ilmawi the Pit Indians. The underground spring and reservoir are the result of all the volcanism in the area. Lava rock is all over the place, and sometimes water percolates through the lava rock and is trapped in underground rivers and reservoirs, or aquifers. One of these aquifers feeds Burney Creek and Burney Falls. Sometimes Burney Creek is dry for 0.5 mile above the falls, but the falls flow year-round, fed by a subterranean source.

Good bicycling is found on the Old Highway Road that runs around the west side of Lake Britton (not CA 89). This road takes off from CA 89 about 0.5 mile south of the McArthur–Burney Falls Memorial State Park entrance. It is a decent ride as far as the now-closed Clark Creek Lodge (a rumored favorite hideout of Al Capone's), but then the road starts climbing earnestly up to CA 89. It's best to turn around at the lodge.

The lovely campsites at McArthur–Burney Falls were constructed by the Civilian Conservation Corps (CCC) in the 1930s. Many of them back into the canyon rim, where a trail heads down to the lake. With plenty of good pitch space, this is prime tent camping.

See how few bushes there are? At first I thought they were pruned by a busy ranger. Not so—a friendly ranger informed me that rainfall on the porous basalt rock quickly soaks too deep for the shallow roots of most bushes—another effect of volcanism. She also gave me some good advice. When making reservations, look for a tent-trailer site. It seems there are 85 tent-trailer sites but only 17 tent sites, so your chances of getting a reservation are vastly improved. Upon arrival, you may ask the ranger to transfer to a tent site if one is available.

If popular McArthur–Burney Falls is full, camp at Northshore, a Pacific Gas & Electric campground just around the lake. This small lakeshore campground (29 sites; walk-in or reservations) always feels peaceful. Like most PG&E campgrounds, Northshore is clean, well run, and beautiful in an understated way. To reach Northshore, just turn left out of the main gate of McArthur–Burney Falls, and drive north on CA 89 around the east shore of Lake Britton. Find Clarks Creek Road (otherwise known as Old Highway Road) on the left, drive 0.9 mile to the entrance on the left, and continue 1 mile down the winding road.

Lake Britton is enchanting. Mist purls down from the hills and spills over the water, and you'll expect a scene from a James Fenimore Cooper novel to materialize before your astonished eyes.

McArthur-Burney Falls Memorial State Park Campgrounds

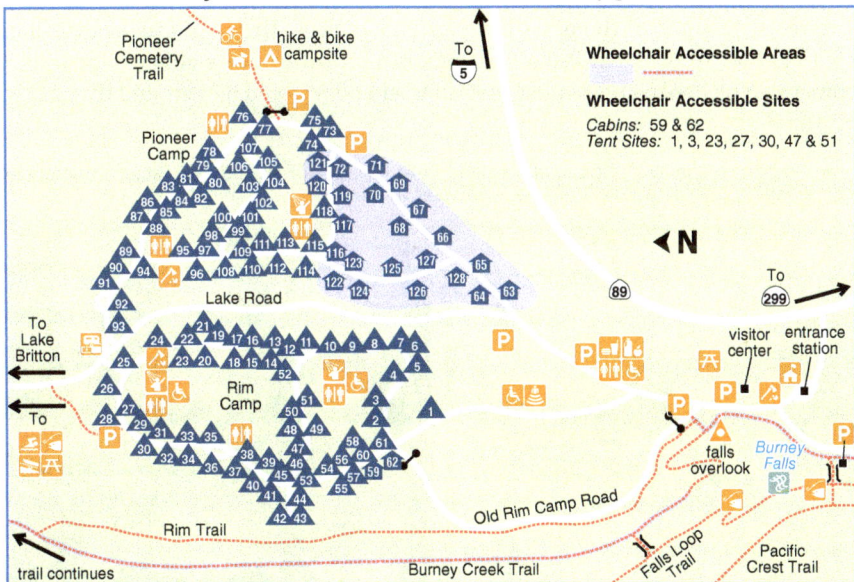

GETTING THERE

From Burney, drive east on CA 299 until it intersects with CA 89. Drive north to the McArthur–Burney Falls Memorial State Park entrance.

GPS COORDINATES: N41° 0.992' W121° 38.948'

26

Mill Creek Falls and Blue Lake Campgrounds

Beauty ★★★★★ / Privacy ★★★★ / Spaciousness ★★★★★ / Quiet ★★★★★ / Security ★★★★★ / Cleanliness ★★★★★

Come to the pristine Warner Wilderness. A bit of a safari, this is the one trip you will never regret.

These two campgrounds are out in the middle of nowhere—the South Warner Wilderness is tucked away in California's northeastern corner. It takes forever to get here, but the drive is stunningly beautiful and well worth the effort. Nowhere in the West do you find an area so pristine and so untrammeled. South Warner is big-sky country.

As fraternal twins often are, Mill Creek Falls and Blue Lake Campgrounds are like day and night. Blue Lake Campground is big and bustling, with a boat launch and plenty of anglers. However, the well-designed campground—like a tiered wedding cake on a high point going out into Blue Lake—gives the campsites a private, secluded feeling. You are separated from your neighbors, and everywhere you look, there are the bright flashes of blue from natural Blue Lake. Come here if you have a boat and want to go fishing (5 miles per hour speed limit).

I talked with some of the other campers and anglers. They had caught their limit of planted rainbow trout but talked about some big brown trout weighing 15 pounds. One old-timer said he hooked one earlier that summer and it towed him around the lake.

Enjoy an "out-there-and-away-from-it-all" experience at Mill Creek Falls and Blue Lake Campgrounds, where the fishing is great in almost any body of water you find.

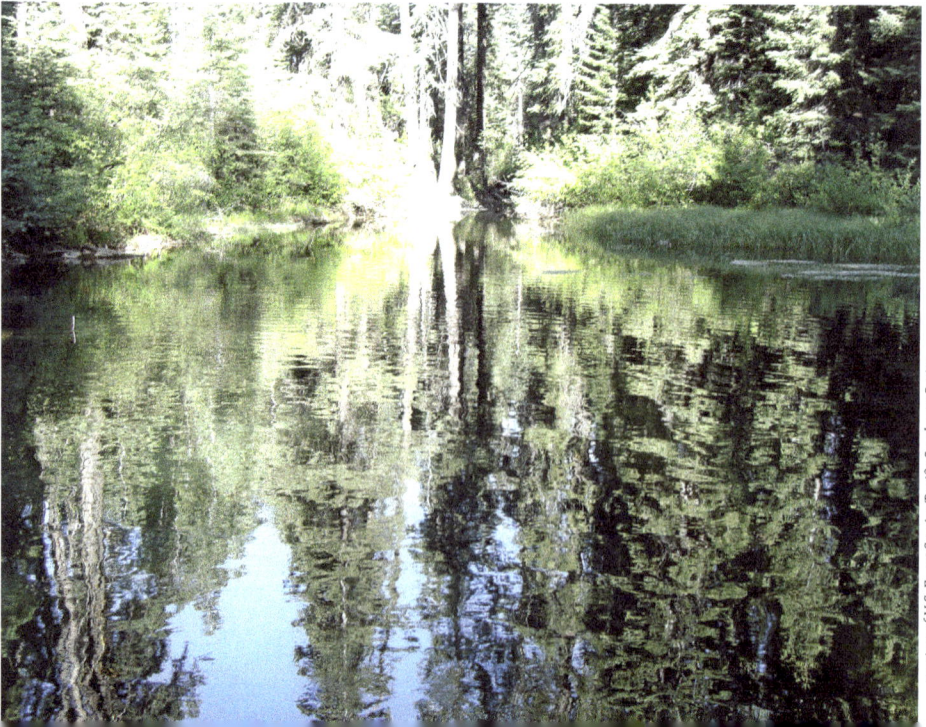

courtesy of U.S. Forest Service/Pacific Southwest Region

KEY INFORMATION

LOCATION: Mill Creek Falls: County Road 64, 11 miles east of I-395 in Eagleville, CA 96110; Blue Lake: Blue Lake Road, 15 miles southeast of I-395 in Madeline, CA 96119

OPERATED BY: Modoc National Forest, Warner Mountain Ranger District

CONTACT: 530-279-6116; www.fs.usda.gov /modoc

OPEN: Mid-May–October, weather permitting (call ahead for weather)

SITES: Mill Creek Falls: 19 sites; Blue Lake: 52 sites

EACH SITE HAS: Picnic table, fireplace

ASSIGNMENT: First come, first served; no reservations

REGISTRATION: By entrance

AMENITIES: Water, vault toilets, boat ramp

PARKING: At individual site

FEE: Blue Lake: $14; Mill Creek: $12

ELEVATION: Blue Lake: 6,000'; Mill Creek: 5,700'

RESTRICTIONS:

PETS: On leash only

FIRES: In fireplace

ALCOHOL: No restrictions

VEHICLES: Mill Creek: RVs up to 22 feet; Blue Lake: up to 30 feet

OTHER: Check weather and water availability; 14-day stay limit

Mill Creek Falls Campground is the best destination in the area for hikers and hiking anglers. A smaller campground, it features sites that are set in a hollow under the pines. It is clean and intimate. The smell of the woods is almost overwhelming. A short walk away (maybe a mile) is Clear Lake. A natural lake, formed by a landslide, it has some big brown trout as well, though not in the same class as Blue Lake. But here you can enjoy solitude, the pines and rocks reflecting off the water, and the nice little jaunt to a place where you won't see or hear the internal combustion engine (although there is no guarantee the U.S. Forest Service won't let them cut around Mill Creek Falls—so write your congressperson!).

To reach Clear Lake, find the trailhead right across from campsite 10 by a parking area. There's a display map, but it's best to come equipped with your own South Warner Wilderness–Modoc National Forest map in case you opt to hike past Clear Lake. With fishing rod in hand, head up the trail. You'll come to a sign pointing left to Mill Creek Falls. It's a 200-yard diversion to admire them. Back on the main trail, carry on to Clear Lake. A trail loop goes left around it. This beautiful lake is close enough to Mill Creek Falls Campground that you can hike up for a quick lunch, or even a sundowner, and still make it back to camp with the last light.

A great fishing hike heads up Mill Creek from the Soup Springs Trailhead. Drive out of Mill Creek Falls Campground, and take a right on West Warner Road. Then take another right on FS 40N24 and find the Soup Springs Trailhead on your right. Hike up over a hill into Mill Creek Valley. Here you will hit Mill Creek and soon will see where it runs into Slide Creek Trail. Go left on the Mill Creek Trail, and head up the left side of Mill Creek for a couple of miles (the fishing here can be quite good). If you are truly ambitious and have the time, continue another 4 miles to the summit of Warren Peak.

The nearest supplies are available in the town of Likely, which has gas, ice, and other basics at the corner store. But if you need meat or groceries, then head on up to Alturas. This place is hopping! Not only does it have the county's only two traffic lights, but it also offers a great museum filled with esoteric exhibits, the wild and woolly Niles Hotel on Main Street, and a supermarket on CA 299.

Mill Creek Falls and Blue Lake Campgrounds

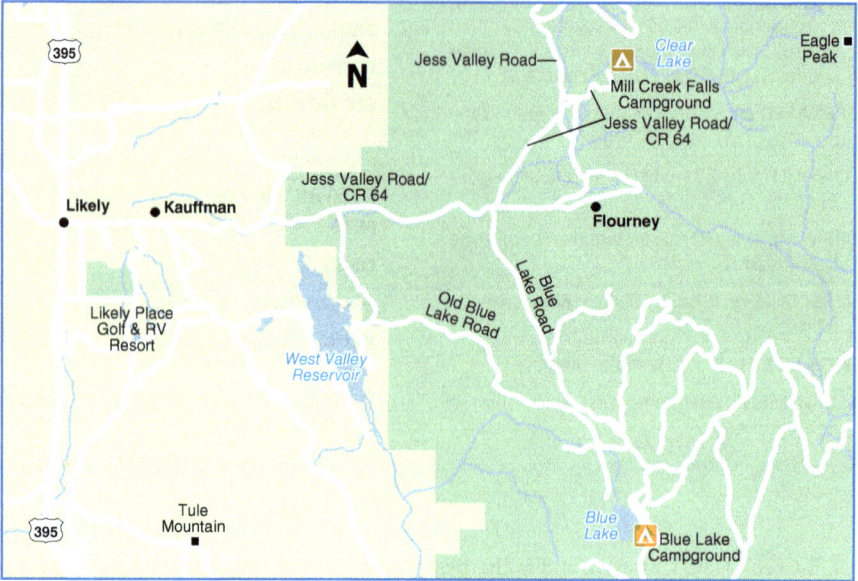

Map labels: 395, N, Jess Valley Road, Clear Lake, Eagle Peak, Mill Creek Falls Campground, Jess Valley Road/CR 64, Likely, Kauffman, Jess Valley Road/CR 64, Flourney, Likely Place Golf & RV Resort, Old Blue Lake Road, Blue Lake Road, West Valley Reservoir, Tule Mountain, 395, Blue Lake, Blue Lake Campground

GETTING THERE

Drive 18 miles south of Alturas on US 395 to Likely. Go left on Jess Valley Road for 9 miles to where the road forks. For Mill Creek, go left at the fork and drive 2.5 miles; bear right and then turn right to stay on County Road 64, and follow the signs to the campground. For Blue Lake, go right at the fork and drive 7 miles on Blue Lake Road to another right turn to stay on Blue Lake Road/CR 510 at South Warner Road. Go 1.7 miles to Blue Lake Campground.

GPS COORDINATES: **BLUE LAKE:** N41° 8.578' W120° 16.808'

MILL CREEK FALLS: N41° 16.600' W120° 17.284'

27

Fowlers Campground

Beauty ★★★★★ / Privacy ★★★ / Spaciousness ★★★ / Quiet ★★★ / Security ★★★★ / Cleanliness ★★★★

Come for the waterfalls; stay for the birding, fishing, and foraging.

As summer heat sizzles off the Central Valley floor, campers and cliff jumpers flock to Lower Falls on the McCloud River like seagulls to an opened bag of chips on the beach. This is river-swimming paradise. The clean, cool, natural spring–fed waters of the Upper McCloud River tumble through a deep basaltic canyon. The result is three dramatic waterfalls within a 1.5-mile stretch. Each waterfall boasts its own deep, aquamarine pool for thick-skinned swimmers who dare brave the year-round, mid-50s temperatures for the thrill of a chill.

Fowlers Campground is central to all three falls and provides campers with excellent river access, a paved hiking trail to the falls, and pretty, shaded sites. Don't forget your field guide and binoculars—the river canyon hosts calliope hummingbirds, Swainson's thrush, and American dippers, as well as willow flycatchers and many other songbirds. This is the ancient happy hunting grounds of the semi-nomadic Winnemem Wintu tribe, who thrived off the bounty of this river canyon prior to the late 1800s. From the land, they foraged for acorns, pine nuts, wild onions, wild plums, chokecherries, mushrooms, elderberries,

Stretch your legs with a short hike to see Upper Falls on the McCloud River. The trail leaves from the campground, passes Middle Falls, and ends at a nice picnic spot at the Upper Falls parking lot.

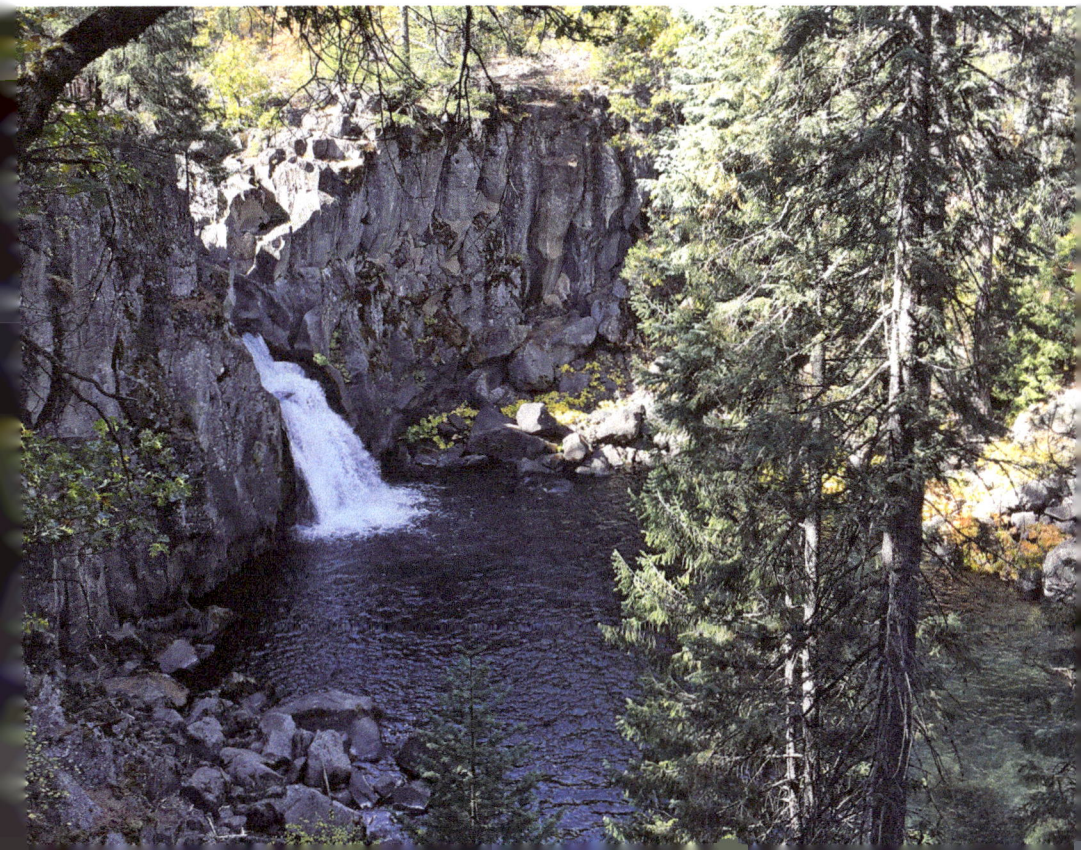

KEY INFORMATION

LOCATION: Fowler Public Camp Road off CA 89, McCloud, CA 96057

OPERATED BY: Shasta-Trinity National Forest, Shasta McCloud Management Unit

CONTACT: McCloud Ranger Station 530-964-2184; www.fs.usda.gov/stnf

OPEN: Third week of April–mid-October

SITES: 35 single sites, 2 double sites

EACH SITE HAS: Picnic table, fire pit

ASSIGNMENT: Online, by phone, or first come, first served (8 sites not reservable)

REGISTRATION: At entrance; reserve at 877-444-6777 or recreation.gov

AMENITIES: Water, vault toilets

PARKING: At individual site

FEE: $15

ELEVATION: 3,400'

RESTRICTIONS:

PETS: Dogs on leash only

FIRES: In fire pit

ALCOHOL: No restrictions

VEHICLES: RVs up to 30 feet

OTHER: 14-day stay limit

currants, watercress, and wild tubers. From the river, they speared fish. In 1874 one traveler reported seeing a group of six Indians spearing 500 salmon in one night. The Wintu spent their summer months camped on the banks above Lower Falls, or Nurunwitipum, as they called it, which means "falls where the salmon turn back."

The once wildly abundant supply of salmon, steelhead, and native trout of the McCloud River isn't near what it was in the 1870s, when white settler T. B. Fowler built a hotel and cottages on the banks where Fowlers Campground now sits. The hotel catered to fisher folk and tourists escaping lowland summer heat until it burned to the ground in the 1930s. In 1943, the resurrection of the Shasta Dam downstream of the Upper McCloud River cut off spawning access for the river's endemic fish species, and so fish populations dwindled. But people still come here to fish. The river is stocked with a robust supply of rainbow and German trout. It's a beautiful fishery: densely forested banks and cool pools offer the perfect habitat for caddis flies; mayflies; and a variety of different stoneflies, including giant salmon flies, golden stoneflies, and little yellow stones. This is fly-fishing heaven, and a number of shops offer guided trips downstream of Lower Falls.

Lower Falls is a pinch in the river where the water drops 15 feet into a large pool. The basaltic cliff banks provide the perfect launchpad for cliff jumpers to take an icy dip. While this swimming hole is within walking distance of Fowlers Campground, it is also accessed by day-use parking, so expect crowds on summer weekends. That just adds to its charm. Come ready to score jumpers as they launch from the park-built diving board, or throw your hat in the ring and take a dip yourself.

My favorite thing to do at Fowlers is walk the river trail to Middle Falls, the most scenic of the three falls, and stare. The trail is short—just about a mile—and you can pick it up right from the campground. Middle Falls is mystical and enchanting, and if you're in the mood for a swim, it's much less crowded than Lower Falls. Middle Falls feels wild, like a step back in time to the days the Wintu speared hundreds of fish a night. Sit on the rocks facing the waterfall and its pool. Bring a journal, a paintbrush, a yoga mat, and a picnic lunch, and soak in the view as the river pours over an 80-foot-wide, 50-foot-tall basaltic cliff. From

Middle Falls, the river trail continues up a short, steep staircase to an overlook of the falls then to 15-foot Upper Falls and a picnic area in the meadow.

When you're not swimming, hiking, birding, or fishing, Fowlers Campground is a nice place to simply enjoy your campsite. The most private campsites are in the lower loop, farthest away from the river. Riverside sites all require a fairly steep hike to get to the actual water, but the sound of the river tumbling through the canyon is the perfect lullaby for a great night's sleep. After a few days at Fowlers, you'll leave feeling refreshed with what the Wintu called *Sau'el mem,* or "sacred water" on the McCloud River.

Fowlers Campground

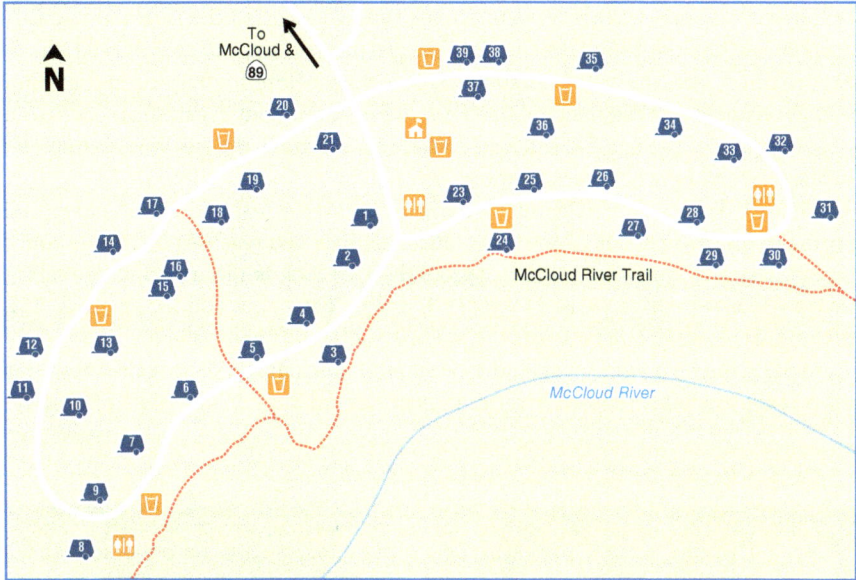

GETTING THERE

From McCloud, go east on CA 89. Drive 5 miles and look for the Fowlers/Lower Falls sign. Turn right just after the sign and drive approximately 1 mile. Once you cross the River Loop Road, take the left fork into the campground. The right fork will take you to the day-use parking area for Lower Falls and the beginning of the River Trail.

GPS COORDINATES: N41° 14.692' W122° 1.396'

28

Hemlock Campground

Beauty ★★★★★ / Privacy ★★★★★ / Spaciousness ★★★★★ / Quiet ★★★★ / Security ★★★★ / Cleanliness ★★★★

A beautiful place to stay in the summer to fish, swim, and enjoy nearby Lava Beds National Monument

The last time my family and I came into Hemlock Campground on Medicine Lake, all we could see were black clouds over the mountain—stretching off as far as Washington state, according to the radio weather reports. By the time we reached the lake, the tule fog was blowing in, with rain not too far behind it. We got our tent up, our gear stowed, the flashlights turned on, and the travel Scrabble game set up before the rain turned to blinding sleet. It blew and blew, then the sleet turned to snow, and we put in earplugs so we wouldn't hear the flapping of the tent fly. After all that, it was morning, the sun was blazing off blue Medicine Lake, and the fish were jumping.

Medicine Lake is beautiful. Hemlock Campground is the first of the three campgrounds you come to on the east side of the lake. After Hemlock you reach A. H. Hogue, and then Medicine Lake. All three are fine campgrounds. Hemlock is more geared to tents, with fewer flat places to park RVs. A. H. Hogue is a little flatter but still favors tents. The flat Medicine Lake Campground attracts the majority of the RVs and trailers.

Hemlock Campground is nearest the beach and boat launch. God knows how, but the beach is composed of actual white sand. It even has a natural kiddie pool, protected by a

Sites at Hemlock favor tent campers over the rest of the crowd.

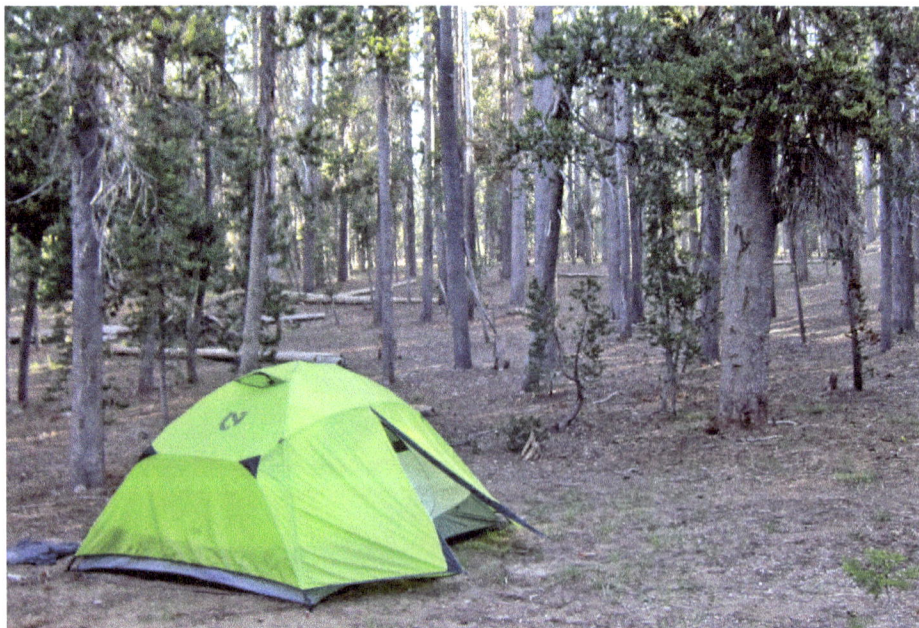

photographed by ex_magician/Flickr.com

KEY INFORMATION

LOCATION: 32 miles east of CA 89 at Bartle, McCloud, CA 96057

OPERATED BY: Modoc National Forest, Doublehead Ranger District

CONTACT: Doublehead Ranger Station 530-667-2246, Modoc National Forest 530-233-5811; www.fs.usda.gov/modoc

OPEN: June–October (depending on road and weather conditions)

SITES: 19 sites for tents or small RVs

EACH SITE HAS: Picnic table, fireplace

ASSIGNMENT: First come, first served

REGISTRATION: At entrance

AMENITIES: Water, vault toilets

PARKING: At individual site

FEE: $14

ELEVATION: 6,700'

RESTRICTIONS:

PETS: On leash only

FIRES: In fireplace

ALCOHOL: No restrictions

VEHICLES: RVs up to 22 feet

OTHER: Don't leave food out; 14-day stay limit. Hemlock Campground is part of the Medicine Lake Recreation Area; all website information is listed under this heading

sandbar. Medicine Lake does allow motorboats, but felicitously, there are specific rules and times for water-skiers and motorboat use (check the current rules posted on the bulletin board). This leaves times when anglers are free to troll for the thousands of trout stocked in the lake every year.

As we found out the hard way, the Modoc plateau has a mercurial nature. Its climate is dry continental, meaning nasty. The weather can change between freezing and sweltering in a whisker. In August titanic thunderstorms on the horizon bring impressive lightning but little rain. In winter the wind blows bitter cold. Pack a bathing suit and a ski jacket. You never know what to expect up here.

This is an incredibly dramatic landscape. No wonder: Hemlock Campground sits atop a 100-square-mile volcano—more massive than Mount Shasta. You don't notice it because the Medicine Lake Highlands come on you as slowly as the curve of the sea. Go see Mammoth Crater, north of Medicine Lake, to look inside the belly of the beast. And Mammoth Crater is not even the mouth of the volcano—that is actually 6 miles south, near Medicine Lake.

Take a couple of hours and hike around Medicine Lake. Include a quick detour on the trail by the Medicine Lake Campground to see Little Medicine Lake. The road past the campgrounds goes halfway around the lake. After that, just follow the lake. You'll find great places to picnic. It's not a bad idea to bring some inclement-weather gear, just in case. Those little pocket raincoats they sell in the camping stores can come in handy. Though little more than a light garbage bag, they are welcome companions when the skies open up.

Glass Mountain, reached via a short hike, is a fun place to visit. Take a right out of Hemlock Campground. Drive south to Forest Service Road 97. Turn left and go 6 miles, passing the first sign for Glass Mountain. Take the second left on FR 43N99. There isn't any real trail; just hike around. Part of this place is privately owned, so mind the signs. What you find here is dacite (gray-colored) and rhyolitic obsidian (sharp and shiny). The Modocs came up here often to gather obsidian to make arrowheads, spearheads, and tools to use and trade with American Indians from as far away as the coast.

Other great hikes await down in Lava Beds National Monument. You have to explore Captain Jack's Stronghold (get the Lava Beds National Monument brochure for the map to the park, and cough up a couple of quarters for the "Captain Jack's Stronghold" Historical Trail brochure). Try to find out how Captain Jack retreated, and follow the trail. The Thomas Wright Trail (white man's folly) is another hour's hike, as is the Schonchin Butte Trail (short but steep). The Whitney Butte Trail is a day trip, so bring lunch and enjoy yourself. You'll end up on the edge of Callahan Lava Flow. In 1969, skeptics accused NASA of filming the lunar landing there. See for yourself.

There are two ways to get to Lava Beds National Monument. Go north on Volcanic Legacy Scenic Byway, which is the bumpy way (17 miles). Or take FR 97 to FR 10 near Timber Mountain Store at Tionesta (36 miles)—the smoother way. They both take about the same time. It's best to take the corduroy road going downhill, then come back the long way and get gas, ice, and cold drinks at the store. The next-nearest supplies are available at the supermarket in Tulelake.

Hemlock Campground

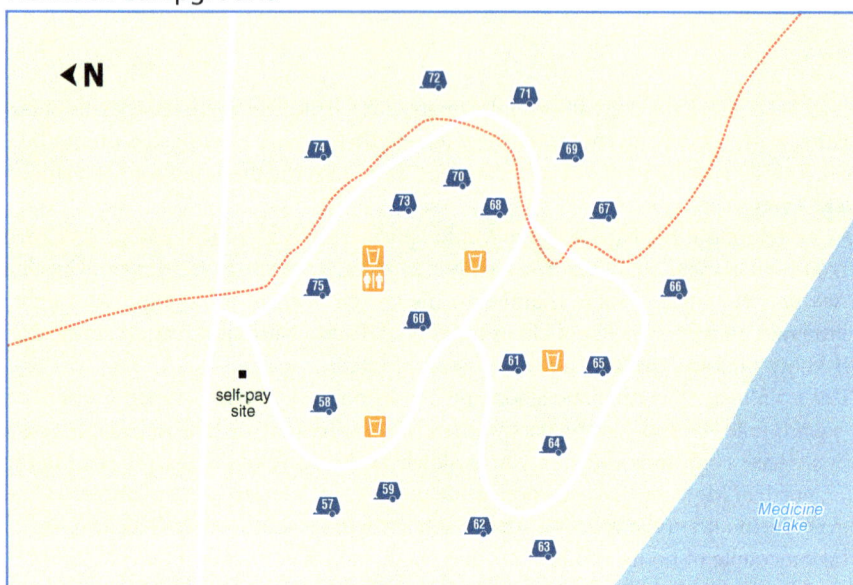

GETTING THERE

From Bartle on CA 89, head northeast up Harris Spring Road/FS 15 for 4.5 miles; veer right onto Medicine Lake Road/FS 49 and continue another 27 miles. Turn left into the Hemlock Campground.

GPS COORDINATES: N41° 35.166' W121° 35.438'

29

Indian Well Campground

Beauty ★★★★★ / Privacy ★★★★ / Spaciousness ★★★ / Quiet ★★★★★ / Security ★★★★★ / Cleanliness ★★★★★

Indian Well is a true destination campground—this is the most awesome spot in Northern California.

For hundreds of years, people have camped on the flat at Indian Well. This is the only level, open ground nearby. Soft pumice covers most of the rocks, so it is easy to pitch a shelter and sleep on the ground. The flat is up high enough that visitors can see for miles. And there's water in the Indian Well Cave, visible by daylight.

The first campers here, the Modoc and their ancestors, lived north of the lava beds along Tule and Lower Klamath Lakes, subsisting on waterfowl, water-lily seeds, and fish and cutting the tule reeds for bedding, hats, and canoes. In the fall, the Modoc camped at Indian Well on their way to the mountains to hunt bear, bighorn sheep, and pronghorn and to harvest manzanita, berries, and pine nuts. The Modoc were fierce and fought with the Pit River people and the Klamath to keep their rich lands. Then settlers came, and the Modoc fought hard against them and the U.S. Army. The Indians lost—Modoc culture was eradicated to make way for ranchers.

Time has marched on, and many of the lakes from which the Modoc fished have been drained; the pronghorn herds are gone; and the bunchgrass the bighorn ate has given way

Vibrant sage and rabbitbrush line the trails, providing shelter for animals across the barren, lava-rock landscape at Indian Well Campground.

KEY INFORMATION

LOCATION: 1 Indian Well Headquarters, Tulelake, CA 96134

OPERATED BY: Lava Beds National Monument

CONTACT: Visitor center 530-667-8113; headquarters 530-667-8100; nps.gov/labe

OPEN: Year-round

SITES: 43

EACH SITE HAS: Picnic table, fireplace, grill

ASSIGNMENT: First come, first served; 1 reservable group site (call 530-667-8113)

REGISTRATION: At entrance

AMENITIES: Water and flush toilets

PARKING: At individual site

FEE: $10, $15 entrance fee/vehicle for 7-day pass

ELEVATION: 4,200'

RESTRICTIONS:

PETS: On leash only

FIRES: In fireplace

ALCOHOL: No restrictions

VEHICLES: RVs up to 30 feet

OTHER: 14-day stay limit

to cheatgrass (an exotic plant from Asia). But we can still come here and camp, explore the Modoc's sacred lava-tube caves, hike among the sage and the rabbitbrush blooming yellow in the fall, and imagine a time when this area was lit only by fire.

Lava Beds National Monument first shocks you then rewards you. The land seems desolate and savage. The lava rocks cut like razors. Then you spot the vegetation and find that the land is rich and full of life. Here the continental plates were pulled apart, so magma rose up from the interior of the earth to form this area. Cinder cones, shield volcanoes, stratovolcanoes, spatter cones, chimneys, pahoehoe lava, and lava-flow caves remain.

I love Lava Beds National Monument. Of all my family's Western trips when I was a child, I remember Lava Beds the best. Even as a little kid, I was awed by the elemental violence that created this land and how quickly the vegetation took over to give life. From the campground, you can hike miles over the rock along Three Sisters Trail. Or drop down into any one of Lava Bed's caves with a flashlight and a map. The whole area is an incredible adventure, and visitors are free to explore responsibly by themselves.

The visitor center, where you can buy the Lava Beds Caves map book, is 0.5 mile from the campground. The park headquarters also lends flashlights if you need to supplement your own. And before you go exploring, you'll need a special cave pass, issued from the visitor center, verifying that your clothes and gear have been screened for fungus spores that could transmit white nose syndrome to the caves' bats. Spores of the cold-loving fungus have been known to hitch a ride on clothes and gear that have been used in other affected caves. As of 2017, the syndrome had not yet made its way to California, and park staff would like to keep it this way.

Going into the caves is no joke. Bring warm clothes (cold air collects in the caves). A hard hat for your head is a good idea, but at least wear a cloth hat. Never go alone, and be sure to tell somebody responsible which cave you are going to explore and when you are going to get back. Gloves, knee pads, a first aid kit, food, and water are musts if you go cave exploring whole hog—most people get bitten by cave exploration and can't stop.

Come prepared for hot and cold camping. Even in the summer, Lava Beds can be cold, and a stiff wind can make a cool day freezing. The dry continental climate of the Modoc Plateau is ferocious, and the interiors of the lava caves are always cold. It can be very dry, so bring lip balm and moisturizing lotion. Bring a good hat with a drawstring to hold it on in the wind. Bring earplugs to use at night so that you won't lose any sleep listening to the tent flapping. Bring shorts and a T-shirt too, because with all the preparation for bad weather, the climate is bound to be balmy on occasion.

Food is unavailable at the visitor center. Buy real food at Tulelake (like a set from *The Last Picture Show*), which actually has a motel. Ice, beer, and hot dogs are available at rustic Tionesta (you have to go a few hundred yards off the road). Don't pass either town without getting gas—they have the only pumps for miles.

Season permitting, try to camp up on the Medicine Lake Volcano, which blew off lava, gas, and cinders for a million years to give us the lava beds. In addition to four campgrounds, there's a good beach, decent fishing, and Mammoth Crater and Glass Mountain.

Indian Well Campground

GETTING THERE

From Tulelake, drive south on CA 139. Before Newell, go right on the Great Northern Road/County Road 111 about 6 miles. Next turn right and continue another 18 miles, first going west on CR 120 and then going south on CR 10, to the Lava Beds National Monument Visitor Center. The entrance to the Indian Well Campground is across from the visitor center.

GPS COORDINATES: N41° 43.034' W121° 30.252'

THE SIERRA NEVADA

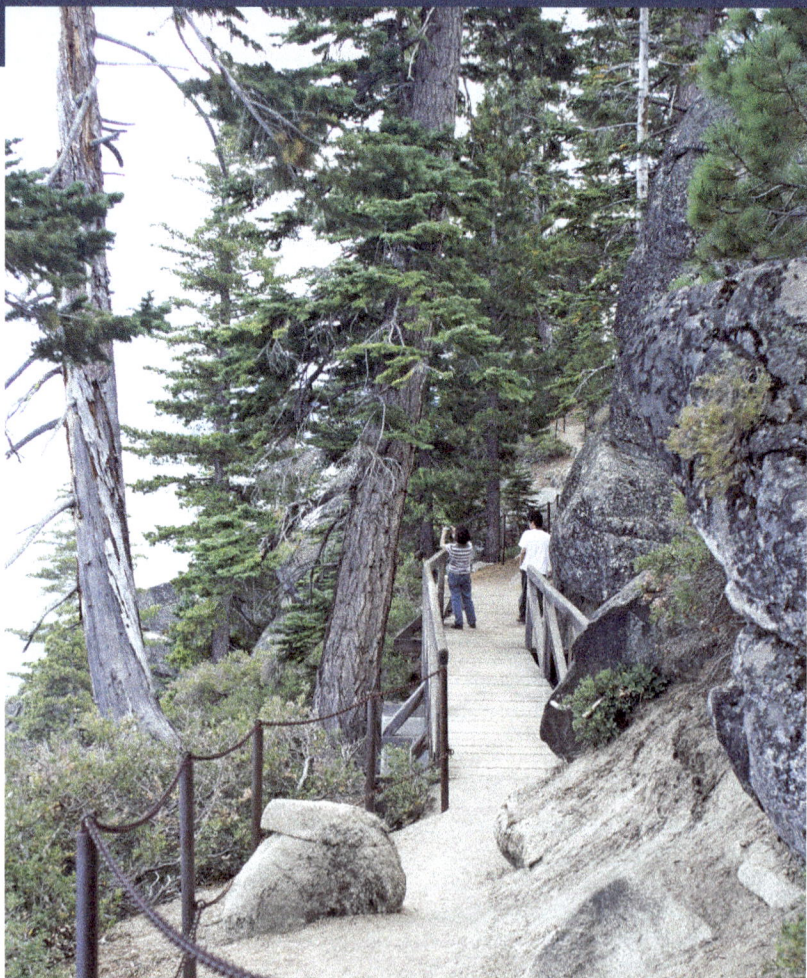

A boardwalk along the Rubicon Trail allows hikers to enjoy views of Lake Tahoe *(see page 141)*.

30

Oak Hollow Campground

Beauty ★★★★ / Privacy ★★★ / Spaciousness ★★★★ / Quiet ★★★ / Security ★★★★★ /
Cleanliness ★★★★★

Open all year, Calaveras Big Trees State Park offers the best camping fall through spring.

In 1852 hungry miners needed red meat. And that's what Augustus T. Dowd was after one fine spring day as he chased a wounded bear up the Stanislaus River. Instead of lunch, he found some of the biggest trees he'd ever seen. Using a string, he measured one of the trees. When he got back to town, the string was found to be more than 100 feet long. The story goes that nobody believed Dowd, and nobody would go with him to see the leviathan trees. Later, Dowd told everybody he had shot a huge bear, and when curious folks straggled after him to see the bear, they saw the Big Tree instead. Pointing to the immense trunk and lofty top, Dowd cried out, "Boys, do you now believe my big tree story? This is the large grizzly bear I wanted you to see. Do you still think it's a yarn?"

Indeed, the Big Tree is an awesome sight. John Muir noted, "The Big Tree is nature's forest masterpiece, and as far as I know, the greatest of living things. It belongs to an ancient stock, as its remains in old rocks show, and has a strange air of other days about it, a thoroughbred look inherited from the long ago—the auld lang syne of trees."

The Big Stump, or Discovery Tree, located near the visitor center on the North Grove Trail in Calaveras Big Trees State Park, measures 25 feet in diameter. This Giant Sequoia was estimated to be 1,244 years old when it was felled in June 1853 by Augustus T. Dowd.

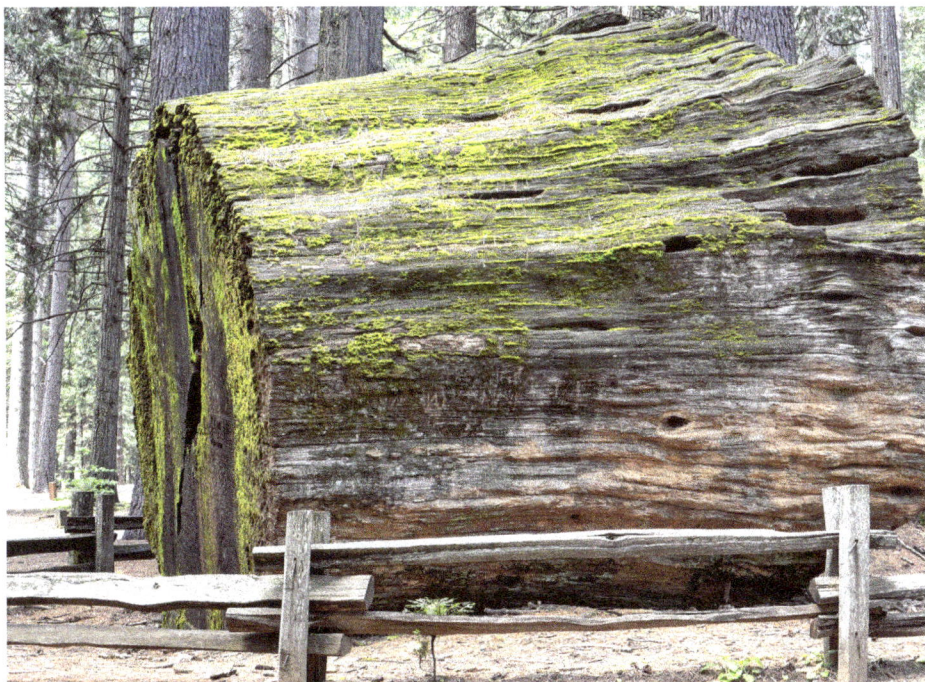

KEY INFORMATION

LOCATION: Big Trees Parkway off CA 4, Arnold, CA 95223

OPERATED BY: Calaveras Big Trees State Park

CONTACT: 209-795-2334; www.parks. ca.gov

OPEN: Mid-May–mid-September

SITES: 34 tent sites, 17 sites for tents or RVs up to 30 feet, 1 wheelchair-accessible site

EACH SITE HAS: Picnic table, fire pit, grate, camp stove

ASSIGNMENT: First come, first served; reservations recommended

REGISTRATION: By entrance; reserve at 800-444-7275 or reservecalifornia.com

AMENITIES: Water, flush toilets, showers, firewood for sale

PARKING: At individual site

FEE: $35, $8 nonrefundable reservation fee

ELEVATION: 4,800'

RESTRICTIONS:

PETS: On leash only, not allowed on trails

FIRES: In fireplace

ALCOHOL: No restrictions

VEHICLES: RVs up to 30 feet, 2 vehicles/site

OTHER: Reservations recommended on holidays and summer weekends; 15-day stay limit; do not feed bears; trees, plants, and animals protected in park

---

Hardly had the forty-niners' wonder faded when they resolved to cut a Big Tree down. They tried axes and saws—nothing doing. Finally they decided to drill with pump augers through to the center from opposite sides. It took five men 22 days to accomplish the job. The tree fell with a crash heard for miles around. Immediately the bark was stripped off and sent to New York City to show the folks the wonders of California. And soon, folks came out to see the Big Trees.

They danced on dance floors made from the stumps. They rode horses through hollowed out Big Tree logs. They bowled on alleys made from the trees. They named the giants fancifully, as in "Pride of the Forest," or after heroes, as in "Washington." They argued over what to call the Big Tree—"Vegetable Monster" was one name in vogue, briefly. But "Sequoia" seems to have won out in the end (after a Cherokee Indian, Sequoyah, who established an alphabet for the Cherokee language). Then they named the Big Tree Grove "Calaveras," after a skull found in some caves nearby—which was probably from an Indian burial.

Now we can camp under the Calaveras Big Trees at North Grove Campground—although the camping is lots better down at nearby Oak Hollow Campground. Never mind that Oak Hollow Campground has no Big Trees. It's a beautiful campground and a good base camp from which to explore the Calaveras South Grove Natural Preserve. At South Grove you have to hike in like Augustus T. Dowd did and earn your marvel by a sensationally lovely but untaxing hike. Drive to South Grove (or bicycle—good bicycling in the park) and park. Cross pretty Beaver Creek—notice the tiny plaques nailed on the end of each bridge board, honoring a park supporter—and head off for the Big Trees.

The park offers a well-written interpretive guide for sale at the trailhead, explaining what visitors see along the way. The last time I visited the South Grove, we double-timed out after seeing the Big Trees and hiked up the fisherman trail alongside Beaver Creek until we found a good place to splash around.

The fishing was good too, as a strapping young lad proved by pulling two chunky trout from his creel for our inspection. He was wading around the creek barefoot and showed us his blue toes after he put away the fish. "Don't feel a thing," he cheerfully exclaimed.

Back at Oak Hollow Campground, the hot, quarter-metered showers are worth every penny. The campsites are nicely arranged, with enough space and brush between them so you don't feel crowded. Between campsites 123 and 124, a trail heads down to the river. Going the other way, you come to the scenic overlook.

Don't forget to see Columbia State Historic Park. A huge hit with kids and adults, this restored gold-rush town offers gold panning, stagecoach rides, mine tours, and cold beer at the saloon.

It is worth it to make a reservation if possible. I always like to camp on the periphery of the campground so the backyard of the campsite is the woods. I also like to be as far away from the campground entrance and the bathrooms as possible. At Oak Hollow, sites 83, 85–86, 90–91, 93–96, 112–113, 123, and 128 are among the best.

Oak Hollow Campground

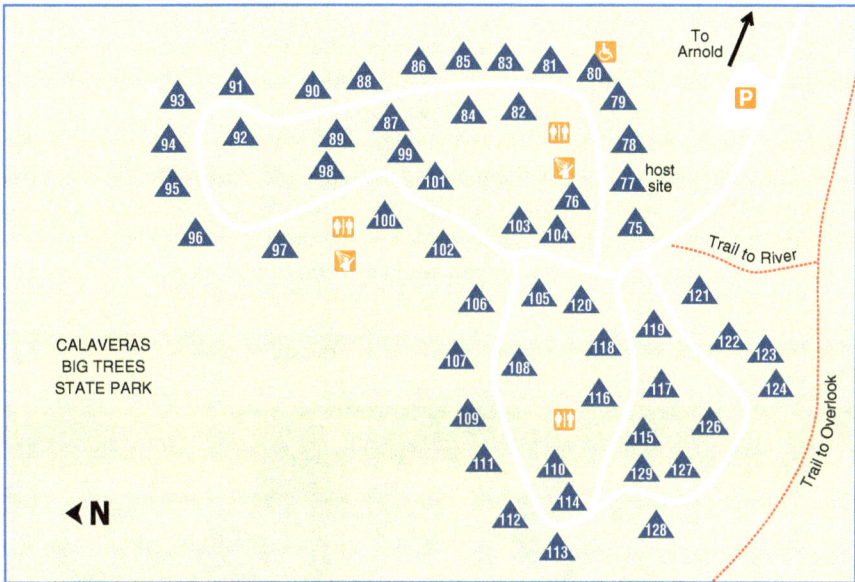

GETTING THERE

From Angels Camp on CA 49, head 26 miles north on CA 4 through Arnold to Calaveras Big Trees State Park. Oak Hollow Campground is a few miles from the park entrance.

GPS COORDINATES: N38° 16.393' W120° 17.450'

31

Wakalu Hep Yo Campground

Beauty ★★★★★ / Privacy ★★★★ / Spaciousness ★★★★ / Quiet ★★★★★ / Security ★★★★★ / Cleanliness ★★★★★

Constructed in 1999, this well-planned campground is nestled in woods above the Stanislaus River.

Wakalu Hep Yo (sometimes spelled Wakaluu Hepyoo) means "wild river" in the American Indian dialect Miwuk. The campground sits on a sloping bank above the Stanislaus River, in woods where the Miwuk people lived seasonally for more than 2,000 years. Wakalu Hep Yo hosts incredibly nice camping yet still preserves historic Miwuk features, including grinding stones and middens. It's a great cultural experience, accentuated by campground signs in both English and Miwuk.

Wakalu Hep Yo would be a wonderful campground even without its location on the Stanislaus River, but the large rushing waterway boosts the camping experience to the upper echelon of California tent pitching. Downslope from the campsites, the river is easily reached by a paved and dirt trail network that threads through the campground. Fishing is popular, and although signs warn about strong currents and drownings, on a hot day it's nearly impossible to resist taking a dip in the pristine, crystal-clear, cool water. Use good sense here: if you want to take the plunge, stick to the deep, placid pools and away from the shallows, where the current is strongest, and keep small children out of the river. Giant

The Stanislaus River provides ample recreation opportunities, including whitewater rafting, kayaking, and excellent fishing.

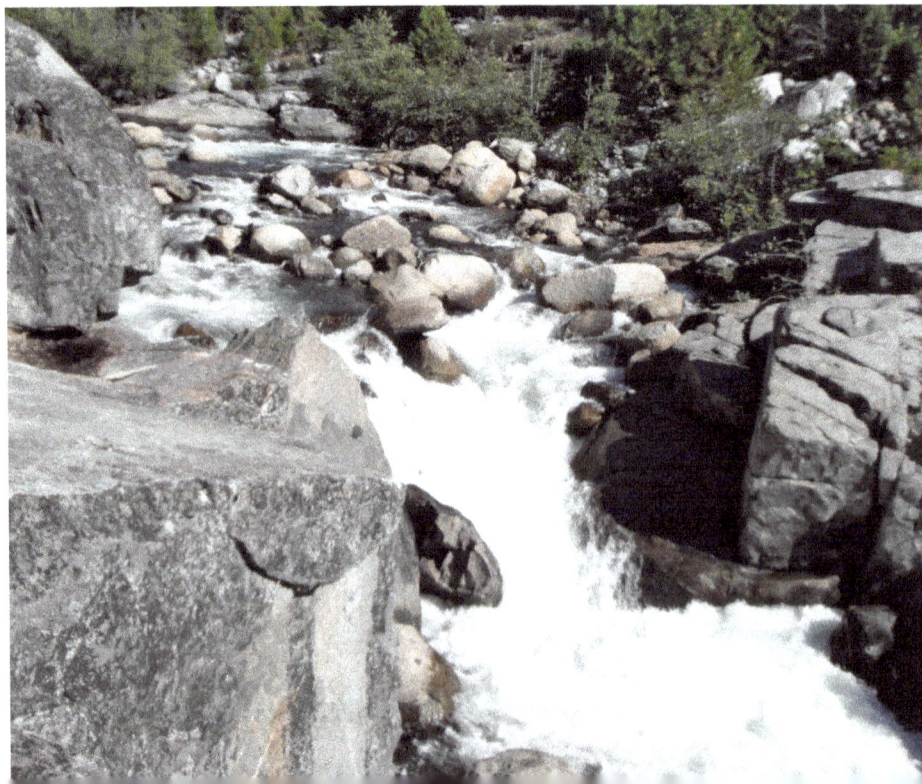

photographed by Lee J. Hahn

KEY INFORMATION

LOCATION: FR 5N02, Arnold, CA 95233

OPERATED BY: Stanislaus National Forest, Calaveras Ranger District

CONTACT: 209-795-1381; www.fs.usda.gov /stanislaus

OPEN: June–October, weather permitting

SITES: 49 total: 27 walk-in sites

EACH SITE HAS: Picnic table, fire ring

ASSIGNMENT: First come, first served; no reservations

REGISTRATION: Self-register at information area near showers, at front of campground

AMENITIES: Flush and vault toilets, hot showers, drinking water

PARKING: At individual site and in small lots for walk-in sites

FEE: $20

ELEVATION: 3,900'

RESTRICTIONS:

PETS: Dogs must be leashed

FIRES: In established pits/rings only

ALCOHOL: No restrictions

VEHICLES: Maximum length 50 feet

OTHER: 14-day stay limit

rock slabs lining the river make perfect spots for basking in the sun. It's a 5-mile, class IV whitewater trip from the raft access at the Sourgrass day-use lot (across the river from the campground) to Calaveras Big Trees State Park (phone the ranger station for current conditions and permit information).

The campground's 49 sites are situated along a balloon-shaped access road. A handful of RV sites sit near the showers at the front of the campground, and the remaining sites are oriented to tents. About half the sites require a walk, ranging from a few steps to a few hundred yards. The remaining sites are the traditional park-and-unpack style, with a few adjacent sites perfect for two families or small groups (the campground limit is six people to a site). All sites have fire pits with grills and big picnic tables. The vegetation in the campground is primarily ponderosa pines, black and live oaks, and cedars. There is little understory vegetation to screen views of the campsites, although some sites are shielded by massive boulders.

With a little effort, you can camp at what we consider the nicest sites, 15 and 16. These require the longest walks but are the closest to the river—perfect if you've come to fish for rainbow and brown trout. The walk-in sites nearest the river offer little privacy but are well spaced. When we camped at Wakalu Hep Yo on a Sunday night in early June, only one of the walk-in sites was occupied. The camp host recommended sites 41 and 42, quiet, shaded sites at the back of the campground loop, but we chose site 33, which required a short walk but provided a big payoff—partial views down to the river and a mixture of shade and sunshine. Because we were partly out of the woods, there was great stargazing on a clear, comfortable night. And in the morning, after three nights of camping, the hot showers (free for campers) were most appreciated.

A very rough fire road departs from the Sourgrass day-use lot on a 2-mile journey to Pine Needle Flat—from our campsite we watched a few four-wheel-drive vehicles struggling back to Boards Crossing Road. Note that the trail is open to hiking, mountain biking, and limited off-highway-vehicle use. For a more sedate hiking experience, make the short drive to the sequoia groves at Calaveras Big Trees State Park. If you want to stretch your legs but not really hike, take an easy stroll through the campground and under the bridge to a lookout above a roaring section of the Stanislaus. The Calaveras Ranger District hosts interpretive programs in the summer months, including basket weaving, Miwuk plant use, and Miwuk songs. Look for grinding stones, bowl-shaped depressions in boulders where Miwuks worked acorns into meal, in the campground—there's one in a fenced area near site 7.

Wakalu Hep Yo is set in a relatively low elevation, unlike the popular campgrounds 20 miles or so farther up CA 4, including the Lake Alpine area, where elevations range from 6,000 to 8,000 feet. Because the temperature drops about three degrees for every 1,000 feet gained, Wakalu Hep Yo is slightly warmer than the campgrounds at Spicer Reservoir and Pine Marten (see page 117). If you're averse to heat, check out Wakalu Hep Yo in autumn.

Arnold and Murphys are the two largest towns on the way to the campground, with grocery and hardware stores, restaurants, gas, and sporting-goods shops (remember you'll need a fishing license if you plan to try your luck for trout). Dorrington and Camp Connell have limited services, but you can pick up ice and other camping staples at Camp Connell's general store. Wine production is steadily increasing in this part of the state, and high-quality vintages from nearby wineries are available, even from the general stores in the area.

Wakalu Hep Yo Campground

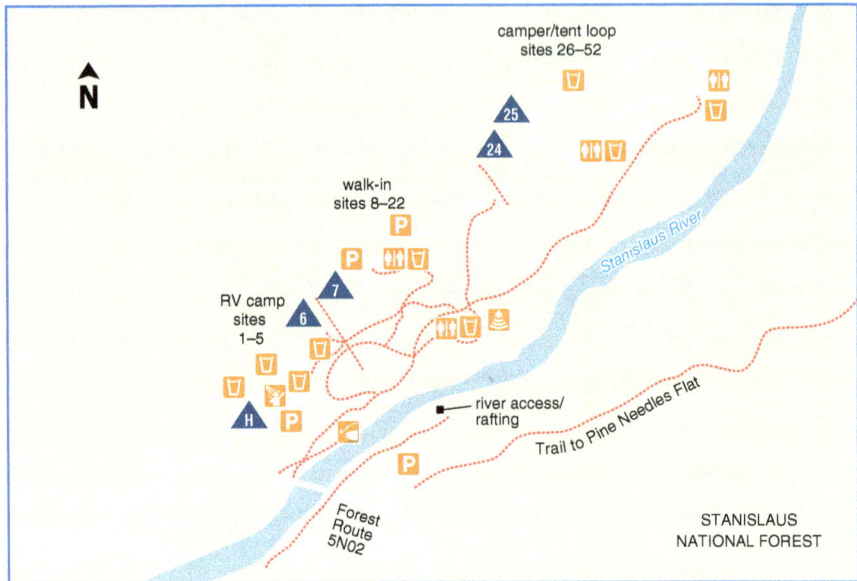

Map of Wakalu Hep Yo Campground showing: N (north arrow), camper/tent loop sites 26–52, sites 25 and 24, walk-in sites 8–22, RV camp sites 1–5, sites 7 and 6, river access/rafting, Stanislaus River, Trail to Pine Needles Flat, Forest Route 5N02, STANISLAUS NATIONAL FOREST.

GETTING THERE

From Angels Camp on CA 49 in Calaveras County, turn east onto CA 4. Drive east 25 miles to the small settlement of Dorrington, then turn right onto Boards Crossing Road. Follow Boards Crossing Road 1.5 miles and veer left onto Forest Service Road 5N02; go about 3.7 miles and then turn right into the campground.

GPS COORDINATES: N38° 19.336' W120° 13.089'

32

Pine Marten Campground

Beauty ★★★★★ / Privacy ★★★★★ / Spaciousness ★★★★★ / Quiet ★★★★ / Security ★★★★★ / Cleanliness ★★★

When the snow melts, Pine Marten Campground is heaven.

Pine Marten Campground is on pretty Lake Alpine below Ebbetts Pass. It is popular, so try to come early on busy summer weekends to get a good site near the water. If you strike out, there are several other campgrounds within rifle shot where you can pitch your tent (there's a ranger station just west of Lake Alpine where you can inquire). It's best to come by Thursday and plan on staying a week. This is prime Sierra Nevada camping.

Ebbetts Pass, just east of Lake Alpine, was named for Major John Ebbetts, who crossed the Sierra Nevada here while looking for a route to build a railroad. He got the nominal credit, but he certainly wasn't the first man to cross here. For tens of thousands of years, American Indians climbed the Sierra Nevada looking for cool weather and food. Their trails went to food sources and summering campgrounds. So when the first gringos tried to follow their trails, they were often frustrated when they found themselves dead-ended at piñon forests and streamside flats.

Rightly, Ebbetts Pass should be named Jedediah Smith Pass because Smith was the first European to make it over the Sierras, in 1827. It was rough going in the snow. "I started with two men, seven horses, and two mules, which I loaded with hay for horses and provisions

Spend the day exploring the many rocky islands in Lake Alpine, an idyllic reservoir on Silver Creek.

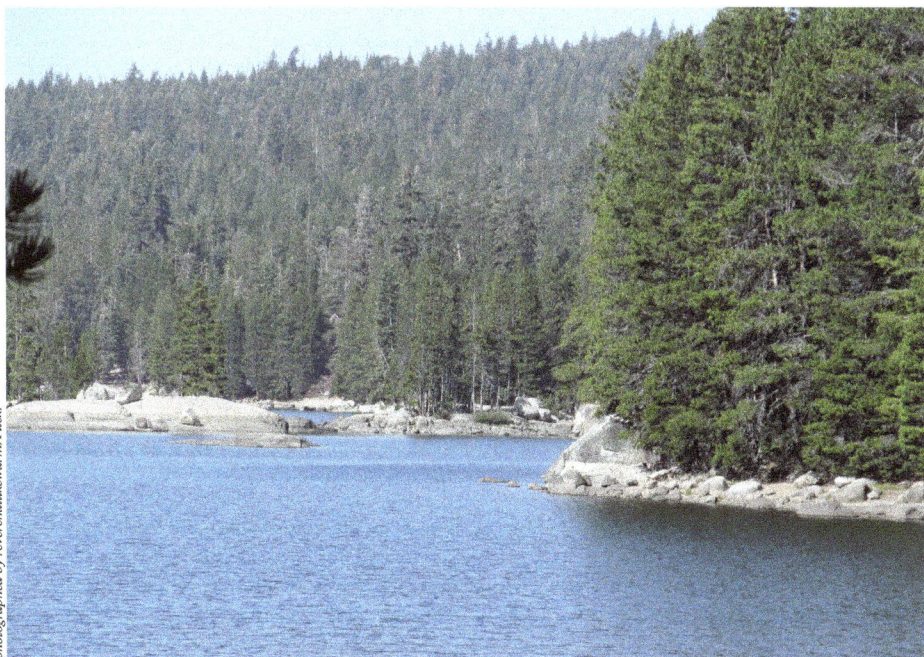

photographed by reverendlukewarm/Flickr

KEY INFORMATION

LOCATION: Alpine State Highway, east end of Lake Alpine, Arnold, CA 95223

OPERATED BY: Stanislaus National Forest, Calaveras Ranger District

CONTACT: 209-795-1381; www.fs.usda.gov /stanislaus

OPEN: June–October (depending on road and weather conditions); opens after last snow; if gate is locked, the grounds are closed

SITES: 32

EACH SITE HAS: Picnic table, fireplace, grill

ASSIGNMENT: First come, first served; no reservations

REGISTRATION: At entrance

AMENITIES: Water; wheelchair-accessible flush and vault toilets

PARKING: At individual site

FEE: $25

ELEVATION: 7,300'

RESTRICTIONS:

PETS: On leash only

FIRES: In fireplace

ALCOHOL: No restrictions

VEHICLES: RVs up to 27 feet

OTHER: Don't leave food out; 14-day stay limit

for ourselves, and started on the 20th of May, and succeeded in crossing it in eight days, having lost only two horses and one mule. I found the snow on the top of the mountain from four to eight feet deep, but it was so consolidated by the heat of the sun that my horses only sank from half a foot to one foot deep." That's from a letter to William Clark—of Lewis and Clark—then superintendent of Indian affairs.

It snows heavily and frequently in this area. In July 1995, the snow drifted 30 feet deep at Pine Marten Campground. Pacific storms sucked in through the Golden Gate head east to the Sierra Nevada below Ebbetts Pass. At about 7,000 feet, the clouds cool down and dump all their moisture as snow.

The last time I camped at Pine Marten Campground, in early June, I found snowdrifts still there. Over the phone, the U.S. Forest Service told me the campground was open. I mentioned this to a Lake Alpine local who remarked, "Well, they don't see much driving around in their fancy pickup trucks, now do they?"

We parked our car in front of the first deep drift and carried our tent and gear into the campground until we found a nice, level, fairly dry spot and pitched the tent. Our drinks went into a drift and I scoured dishes with snow.

A good hike out of Pine Marten Campground is to Inspiration Point. It gets steep in places, but you can get there and back in an hour or so. Pick up the trail just past the Pine Marten Campground entrance. There's a trailhead sign for Inspiration Point–Lakeshore Trail. Follow it through the lodgepoles until you start to climb. The slopes are steep and made of weird stuff called lahar, which was left by volcanic mudflows. The views are spectacular.

Up top, we sat down on a rock and ate a pound of sweet cherries we'd bought in the farmland below and gazed at Lake Alpine basin. It looked like a perfectly natural mountain lake. But looks are deceiving—Pacific Gas & Electric dammed up Silver Creek to make Lake Alpine.

The next day we went fishing in a rented boat but had no luck. I got a lesson from the previously mentioned local about how to affix my worm to the hook. He also asserted that using half a nightcrawler worked better than the whole worm.

It didn't matter anyway. Lake Alpine is gorgeous. There are islands of pines and gray rock—lots of trout for other people to catch, and warm rock to lie on while looking up at the clear cerulean sky. There are hot showers at the resort, as well as a great little bar and restaurant. Rent a boat and explore the shoreline. Hike up the mountains, come back, and jump into the water. It doesn't get any better than this.

Pine Marten Campground

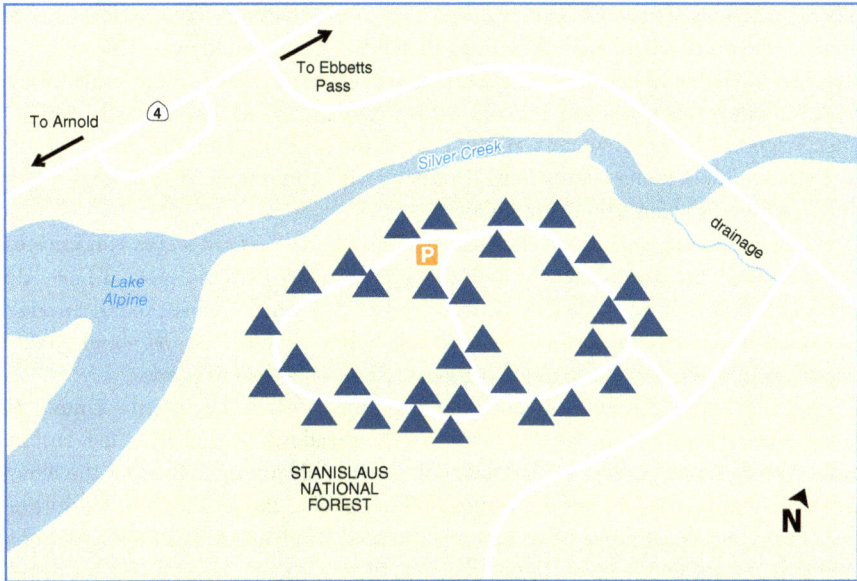

GETTING THERE

From Arnold, drive 29 miles north on CA 4, past Calaveras Big Trees State Park, to Lake Alpine (the town and lake) and the campground entrance on the right just past both of them.

GPS COORDINATES: N38° 28.862' W119° 59.378'

33

Highland Lakes Campground

Beauty ★★★★★ / Privacy ★★★★★ / Spaciousness ★★★★★ / Quiet ★★★★★ / Security ★★★★★ / Cleanliness ★★★★★

Come prepared to stay—this is my favorite Sierra Nevada campground.

This campground is my favorite campground in the Sierra Nevada. At 8,600 feet, the campsites are by the pretty Highland Lakes, in a valley full of bright wildflowers. If you can get in on the road to Highland Lakes, it means the snowdrifts have melted. If the snowdrifts have melted, you know the wildflowers are out—this is a short season. To the north, even in late August, Folger Peak has snowfields. Hiram Peak to the south is as big and brown as a warm bear. There are hikes going everywhere. This is off the beaten track. You don't just happen to show up there, so plan to stay for a while.

The Highland Lakes are up on the west side of Ebbetts Pass. This area is notorious for snow; some years the pass is snowed in until August. In July 1995 the snow at Lake Alpine, a thousand feet farther down, drifted 30 feet deep. Pacific storms get sucked in through the Golden Gate and head east to the Sierra Nevada below Ebbetts Pass. At about 7,000 feet, the clouds cool down and dump all their moisture as snow—lots of snow.

It's not much easier going now until the drifts melt. When they do, the county plows the road, the days get warm, flowers bloom in the meadows, and planted fish run in the streams. The dirt road in off CA 4 is rough going but easily managed by even the wimpiest of sedans. Just go slowly and mind the bumps. It takes off to the southeast just 1 mile below Ebbetts Pass (14.5 miles above Lake Alpine). The road (Highland Lakes Road) goes down a steep hill then runs along pretty Highland Creek, filled with wonderful places for dispersed camping if you have the requisite permit (free at any ranger station) and a bucket and shovel

At the base of 9,706-foot Folger Peak, the Highland Lakes give campers a good sense of high alpine lake camping at the top of the Pacific Crest.

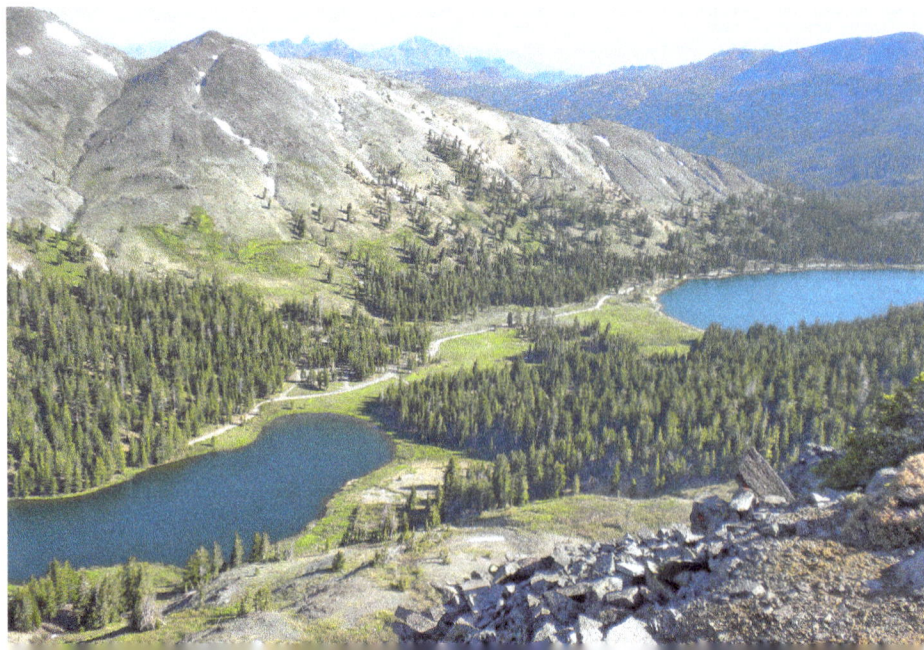

photographed by Douglas Smith

KEY INFORMATION

LOCATION: Highland Lakes Road, 7 miles off CA 4, Arnold, CA 95223

OPERATED BY: Stanislaus National Forest, Calaveras Ranger District

CONTACT: 209-795-1381; www.fs.usda.gov /stanislaus

OPEN: Late June–October (weather permitting)

SITES: 35 sites for tents

EACH SITE HAS: Picnic table, fireplace

ASSIGNMENT: First come, first served; no reservations

REGISTRATION: At entrance

AMENITIES: Hand-pump well water, vault toilets

PARKING: At individual site

FEE: $12

ELEVATION: 8,600'

RESTRICTIONS:

PETS: On leash only

FIRES: In fireplace

ALCOHOL: No restrictions

VEHICLES: Large RVs or trailers not recommended

OTHER: Don't leave food out; 14-day stay limit

for fire suppression. Some of the area is designated Rehabilitation Project, meaning you can walk in, carry in a tent, and camp, but you can't drive your vehicle in. Of course, where it is not posted, you can drive in on existing access roads and camp by your car.

Pass fields of purple lupine and crazy shooting stars. After a steep climb, there are the two Highland Lakes and the lower part of the campground, on the right under lightning-blasted pines. The sites are not well designed, but they are pretty and clean. There's one outhouse near the middle of camp, and a pump for water across from site 10. Remember to bring a bucket for hauling water from the pump to your campsite.

To reach the upper part of the campground, take the dirt road that goes west between the two lakes. It has a confusing sign that appears to advise four-wheel-drive only; ignore this. The road to the camp area (only a few hundred yards long) is just like the road you drove in on. Any sedan can make it easily. These sites are just above the lakes in a stand of pines. Right away, you'll see the pump and outhouse. The campsites are back in under the pines and a short walk from Upper Highland Lake. If you want privacy, camp up here. If you have kids who want to run around, or if you like the western sun to warm your bones, camp in the Lower Highland Lake area below, where it is sunnier and flatter.

Bring supplies. The nearest store is at Lake Alpine or east to Markleeville. Bring an extra cooler filled with ice, and duct-tape the top. Leave coolers in the shade. Put a wet cloth over the coolers and let evaporation cool the outsides. Consider buying a collapsible cooler for extra storage. Bring water shoes for the lake. Think about bringing a little inflatable boat (at chain stores everywhere for $50 or less) to float around in with a book and fishing gear (brook trout). Buy a Lake Alpine–Carson-Iceberg Wilderness map online or at the ranger station so you can navigate the trails around the lakes. (Or buy the more ambitious U.S. Forest Service map at any nearby ranger station.) Remember sunscreen, as the air is thin and the sun strong. You'll also want lip balm and moisturizing lotion, as it is dry. Bring cotton balls if the kids tend to have nosebleeds. Borrow from the other campers if you forget anything—most campers are friendly and are willing to help by lending things that they prudently remembered to bring along.

Camping at Highland Lakes Campground requires a little extra forethought and travel time, but it's worth it. Remember, call ahead to get road conditions, to find out whether the campground is open, and to see if drinking water is available. If there is no drinking water, boil lake water (5 minutes at a rolling boil), or buy a water filter from a camping store.

Highland Lakes Campground

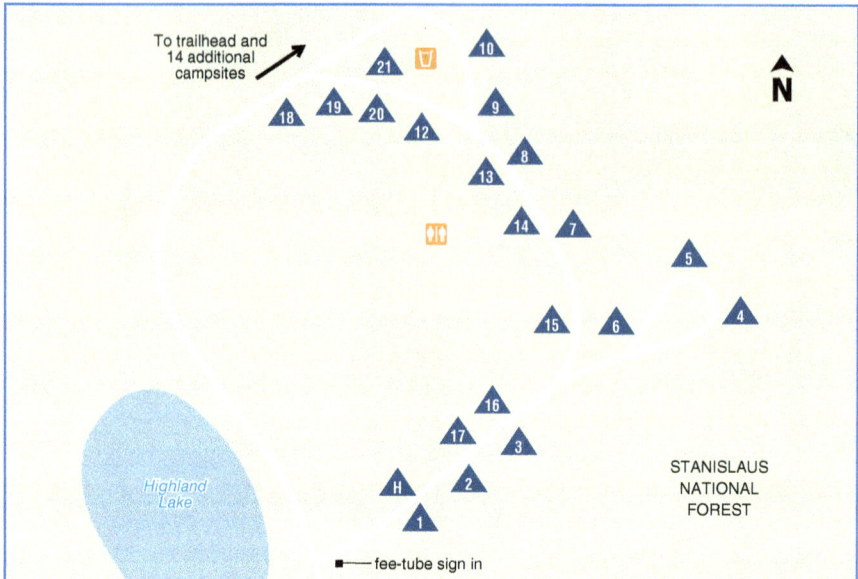

GETTING THERE

From Arnold, go 29 miles east on CA 4 to Lake Alpine. Continue 15 miles past Lake Alpine Resort to Highland Lakes Road (signed to Highland Lakes) on the right. At this point, you will be 1 mile west of Ebbetts Pass. Drive 7.5 miles in on a graded dirt road.

GPS COORDINATES: N38° 29.312' W119° 48.410'

34

Silver Creek Campground

Beauty ★★★★★ / Privacy ★★ / Spaciousness ★★★★★ / Quiet ★★ / Security ★★★★★ /
Cleanliness ★★★★

Silver Creek Campground makes you feel the massive Sierra Nevada.

Camping at Silver Creek Campground is like sleeping on the shoulder of a huge beast: the Sierra Nevada, which is a huge hunk of granite thrust from the earth. It is tilted so the western slope is gradual, while the east side rises almost straight up. Silver Creek Campground hangs on just below the 8,730-foot Ebbetts Pass. The campground is on a piece of land like the prow of a ship, with Ebbetts Pass Road running down the center. The north side of the campground has Silver Creek on its flank; the south side, Noble Creek. The campsites are well engineered and clean—scoured by the winter and the dry desert air from below.

American Indians came up both sides of the Sierra Nevada in the summer to escape the heat. It was easy to walk up over the pass and visit with folks from the other side. Yokuts from the west traded deer, antelope, and elk skins; baskets; acorns; and seashells for piñon nuts, red paint, strong bows backed with sinew, pumice stones, and obsidian from the Paiute on the east.

Hike along Noble Creek to reach the Pacific Crest Trail, or fish along Silver Creek at Silver Creek East Campground.

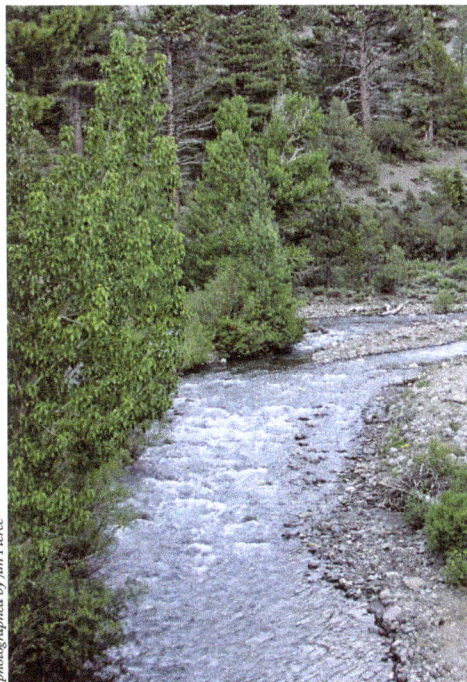

photographed by Jim Pierce

The first white man to attempt the Sierra Nevada crossing was Jedediah Strong Smith. He came through California from the south with a band of trappers in 1826. Looking for beaver in the streams running down out of the Sierra Nevada, Smith noted "a great many Indians, mostly naked and destitute of arms, with the exception of bows and arrows, and what is very singular among Indians, they cut their hair to the length of three inches. They proved to be friendly. Their manner of living is on fish, roots, acorns, and grass."

Eager to get back to rendezvous at the Great Salt Lake, Smith and his men failed two attempts to cross going up the Kings River and the American River. Finally, Smith led his men up an Indian path along the Stanislaus River and over the mountains, near what is now called Ebbetts Pass. They arrived at the Great Salt Lake with only one horse and a mule. They had eaten the rest of their livestock along the way.

KEY INFORMATION

LOCATION: 12.3 miles south of Markleeville, CA 96120 on CA 4, east of Ebbetts Pass

OPERATED BY: Humboldt-Toiyabe National Forest, Carson Ranger District

CONTACT: 775-882-2766; www.fs.usda.gov/htnf

OPEN: Mid-June–mid-September (weather permitting)

SITES: 22 sites for tents and RVs

EACH SITE HAS: Picnic table, fire ring

ASSIGNMENT: Some sites are reservable; others are first come, first served

REGISTRATION: At entrance; reserve at 877-444-6777 or recreation.gov

AMENITIES: Water, vault toilets, food locker

PARKING: At individual site

FEE: $18, $9 nonrefundable reservation fee

ELEVATION: 7,100'

RESTRICTIONS:

PETS: On leash only

FIRES: In fire ring

ALCOHOL: No restrictions

VEHICLES: RVs up to 35 feet

OTHER: Don't leave food out

At Silver Creek Campground, watch the stars move across the night sky and imagine you're on the deck of a huge ship—this hunk of granite that slides across the earth over the hot magma below. From time to time, a lone car's lights come down the pass. You'll feel the power of the mountains and sense the fear of the drivers, the inadequacy of their mechanical conveyances, and the coming snow, which will stop them all dead in their tracks. Old Jedediah Smith must have felt that way—awed, far from home, and scared to death.

A good day hike from camp is up Noble Creek to Noble Lake. Noble Creek is the stream by the south campground area. Follow the stream up the mountain until you meet the Pacific Crest Trail. Go left on the trail and zigzag up through the granite and sage. When you reach the top, Noble Lake is off to the right. What a beautiful spot! To my companions' horror, I actually jumped in and took a dip in the gelid water.

A less rigorous way to reach Noble Lake (although still a day hike) is to drive up to the top of Ebbetts Pass. Park at the summit or a couple hundred yards down the pass toward Silver Creek Campground, where there is a turnoff. The Pacific Crest Trail is marked. Head out under the pines. When I was last there, there was a bumper crop of lupine. Hike up through the mule ear, then down toward Noble Canyon and Noble Creek, through the hemlocks and pines to where the Noble Creek Trail from the campground hits the Pacific Crest Trail. From there, you just climb up to the top of Noble Canyon and see Noble Lake on the right.

A shorter hike is into Upper Kinney Lake. This is about 4 miles round-trip and takes off a couple hundred yards east of Ebbetts Pass. Find the Pacific Crest Trail sign on the north side of the road, which is where you'll start hiking. You'll see Lower Kinney Lake on the right then find a split in the trail signed for Upper Kinney Lake; go left and find Upper Kinney Lake. This is a great place to spend the day. The hiking is easy (round-trip should take about 2 hours), and I saw an angler actually pull a nice-sized trout from the lake.

Many folks who stay at Silver Creek Campground are there for the fishing on Silver Creek and down on the Carson. Markleeville is convenient for supplies, and it has a cute little museum. There's Grover Hot Springs State Park just west of Markleeville, with a swimming pool and hot springs, which are open for a small fee. You can also go the other way, west of Ebbetts Pass, and visit Upper and Lower Highland Lakes, or head farther west to Lake Alpine. (Upper and Lower Highland Lakes and Lake Alpine appear in the entry for Highland Lakes Campgrounds, page 120.)

Silver Creek Campground

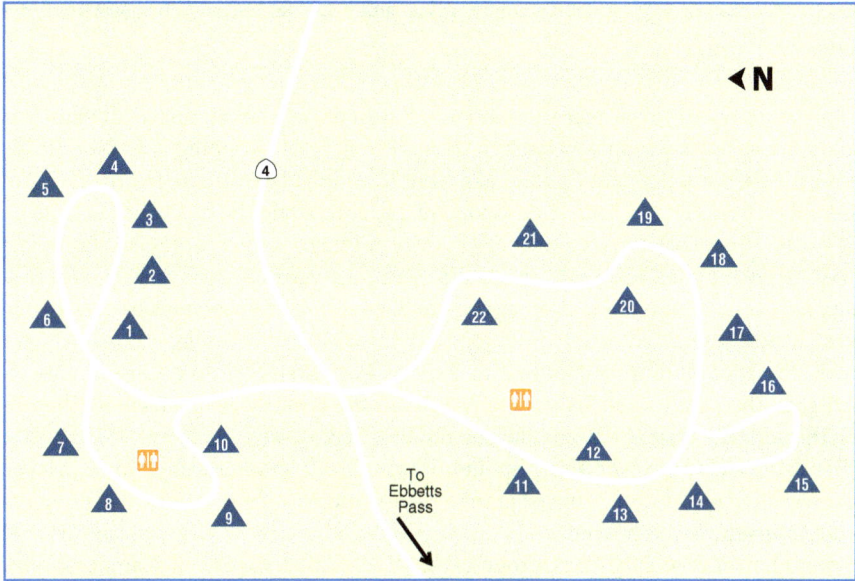

GETTING THERE

From Markleeville, go 5 miles east on CA 89, then stay straight to continue 8 miles west on CA 4 to the campground. From Arnold, drive 48 miles east on CA 4 (over Ebbetts Pass) to the campground.

GPS COORDINATES: N38° 35.297' W119° 47.162'

35

Blue Lakes Campgrounds

Beauty ★★★★★ / Privacy ★★★★★ / Spaciousness ★★★★★ / Quiet ★★★★★ / Security ★★★★★ / Cleanliness ★★★★

Come to Blue Lakes with a week's worth of ice and supplies because you won't want to go home.

Head up Blue Lakes Road near Carson Pass, but make certain you have all your ice and supplies because it's a long way back to town. The nearest shopping is at Woodfords, or up over the pass and down at Caples Lake—but they don't have much. For the first 7 miles off CA 88 (scenic Carson Pass Highway), you'll breeze along the nicely paved Blue Lakes Road by the West Fork Carson River. Then the road turns to dirt for the last bone-jarring 5 miles to Lower Blue Lake. This poor old road gets washed out every spring, and the county has to go in and blade it up again. You'll pass lots of dusty guys in old-style Jeeps looking happy (there's some good off-road driving on Deer Valley Jeep Road, which cuts through the Mokolumne Wilderness to Ebbetts Pass Road, and on Summit City Road, which goes through to Red Lake on CA 88). All the scenery is spectacular. Then you'll come through the dust and pines and see the Blue Lakes.

The Blue Lakes have everything but motorboats: trout, granite islands you can swim to, meadows full of wildflowers, rugged granite ridges, and clear-blue water cold enough to ice down a six-pack. This is heaven.

I ogled Lower Blue Lake Campground and Middle Creek Expansion Campground, then inspected Upper Blue Lake Dam Campground, above the dam, before finally deciding to set up camp at Upper Blue Lake Campground. Why? I don't like to camp below a dam. This is earthquake country, after all.

Hiking opportunities abound near Blue Lakes Campgrounds, with the Pacific Crest Trail in one direction and the steep Deadwood Peak cirque (pictured) in the other.

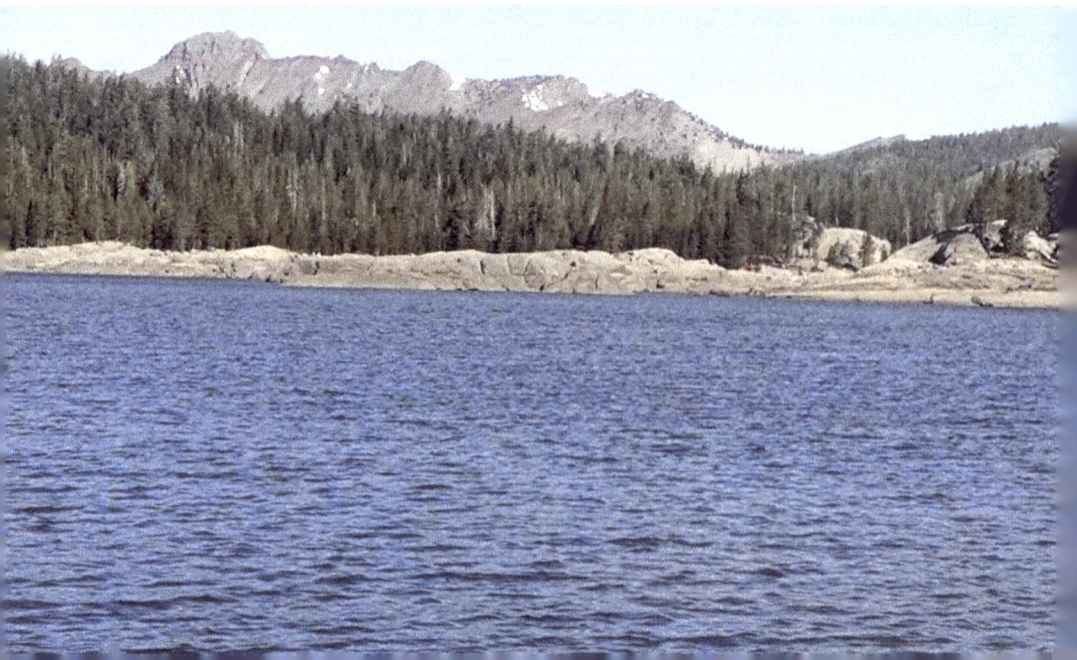

KEY INFORMATION

LOCATION: Blue Lakes Road, 12 miles south of CA 88 at Hope Valley, Markleeville, CA 96120

OPERATED BY: Eldorado National Forest, Amador Ranger District; American Land & Leisure (concessionaire); Pacific Gas & Electric

CONTACT: 209-295-4251; www.fs.usda.gov /eldorado; carsonpass.com/lodging/blue _lakes_camping.html

OPEN: End of May–September (depending on road and weather conditions)

SITES: Upper Blue Lake: 32 sites; Upper Blue Lake Dam: 25 sites; Middle Creek Expansion: 34 sites; Lower Blue Lake: 16 sites

EACH SITE HAS: Picnic table, fireplace

ASSIGNMENT: First come, first served; no reservations

REGISTRATION: At entrance

AMENITIES: Water every third site, vault toilets

PARKING: At individual site

FEE: $2–$24; additional charge for extra vehicles or pets

ELEVATION: 8,200'

RESTRICTIONS:

PETS: On leash only

FIRES: In fireplace

ALCOHOL: No restrictions

VEHICLES: RVs and trailers up to 34 feet (difficult road)

OTHER: Don't leave food out

One day in March 1872, at 2:30 a.m., a monster quake hit the Owens Valley. Felt as far east as Salt Lake City, as far north as Canada, and as far south as Mexico, it shook old John Muir over in Yosemite Valley. He wrote: "I was awakened by a tremendous earthquake, and though I had never enjoyed a storm of this sort, the strange thrilling motion could not be mistaken, and I ran out of the cabin, both glad and frightened, shouting, 'A noble earthquake! A noble earthquake!' feeling sure I was going to learn something."

I want to learn something, but I don't want to get that wet. And, fortunately, both Upper Blue Lake Dam Campground and Upper Blue Lake Campground allay all the worries of the earthquake-conscious camper. Previously, we camped up at Upper Blue Lake Campground, figuring that the campground farthest from the dam was bound to be better. I think it still is, but recently Pacific Gas & Electric, which operates the camp, replaced the water system and had to cut a few trees and reditch for the plumbing.

There's plenty of hiking to be had around the campground, with wildflowers and little unnamed lakes beckoning exploration in the summertime. My family found flowers. There is a meadow just around the northwest side of Upper Blue Lake that was in spectacular bloom. We saw lupines, bachelor's buttons, forget-me-nots, shooting stars, buttercups, yellow snapdragons, swamp lilies, little pink button flowers, Virginia bluebells, penstemon, mule ears, fireweed, and more.

By the campground, the water is shallow and good for swimming. I hiked down through the dwarf mountain willow (deciduous and growing all over the place) and walked out into the water far enough to swim. Remember to bring shoes for wading. Even more great fun would be a cheap inflatable boat to loll about in, arms flung overboard, face to the warm sun.

People were pulling up fish all over the place. The best luck on Upper Blue was above the dam, from the shore. I saw people trolling the deep waters of Lower Blue where Middle Creek runs down from the dam, and I heard somebody bragging about his catch up at Grouse Lake. A path heads to Grouse from a trailhead below Upper Blue Lake Dam.

It is also possible to access the Pacific Crest Trail. On your way in from CA 88, you will pass the trailhead before you get to Lower Blue Lake. You can go either way, although I hear the climb up toward Carson Pass is a bear. You can also access the trail by hiking up the Summit City Road above Upper Blue Lake Campground. Look for an off-road trail on the right that will take you up a ridge to Lost Lakes and the Pacific Crest Trail.

I loved Upper Blue Lake Campground. The pit toilets were immaculate. They even had those paper toilet-seat covers, which really pleased my hygiene-conscious sister.

Blue Lakes Campgrounds

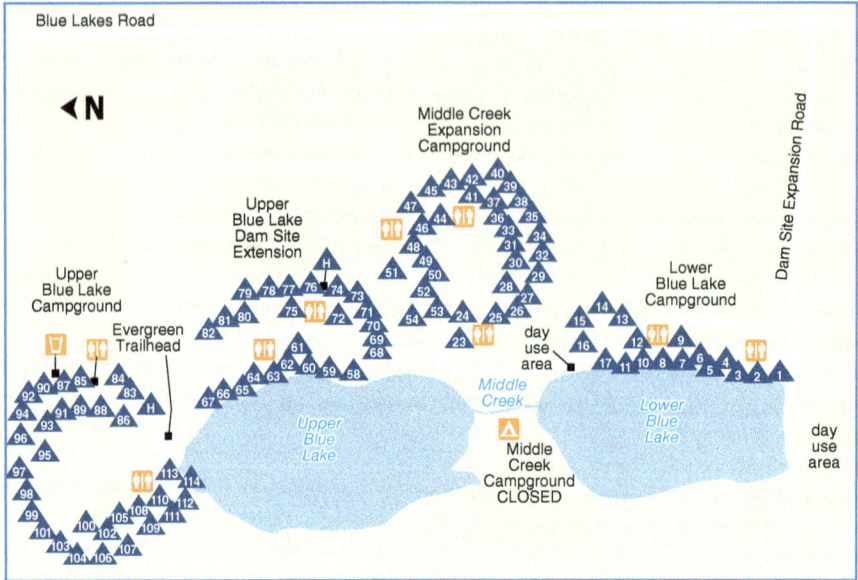

GETTING THERE

From Woodfords, take CA 88 west 9 miles, then turn left on Blue Lakes Road and continue 12 miles. First you will see Lower Blue Lake Campground, then Middle Creek Expansion, Upper Blue Lake Dam, and Upper Blue Lake Campgrounds.

GPS COORDINATES: **UPPER BLUE LAKE:** N38° 38.308' W119° 57.337'
UPPER BLUE LAKE DAM: N38° 37.778' W119° 56.347'
MIDDLE CREEK EXPANSION: N38° 37.595' W119° 56.213'
LOWER BLUE LAKE: N38° 36.719' W119° 55.571'

36

Silver Lake East Campground

Beauty ★★★★★ / Privacy ★★★ / Spaciousness ★★★ / Quiet ★★★ / Security ★★★ / Cleanliness ★★★★

A good place to bring kids, who will entertain each other while you relax.

Silver Lake is a great place to bring a family. With resorts and another big campground nearby, there are always enough kids running around to entertain your own. The lake is a short walk away, where the kids congregate on the shore, and back at the campground the big boulders under the red firs draw youths like bees to honey. While the kids are off playing, you can sit around and take it easy. It's prime camping.

And this area is beautiful. "Nothing in nature I am sure can present scenery more wild, more rugged, more bold, more romantic, and picturesquely beautiful than this mountain scenery." That's how one early pioneer described it. Now CA 88 is the Carson Pass Road, and it was Kit Carson who led Captain John Fremont, with his bodyguard of Delaware Indians, to the crest in 1844.

But it was the Mormon Brigade who engineered the wagon road. In fact, three of them died in an American Indian attack at Tragedy Springs, just southwest of Silver Lake. They were found naked in a shallow grave. The Indians probably killed them for their clothes. It is thought that many were inordinately fascinated with European clothing

Beautiful Silver Lake is part of a string of lakes, called paternosters, which were formed by glacial activity.

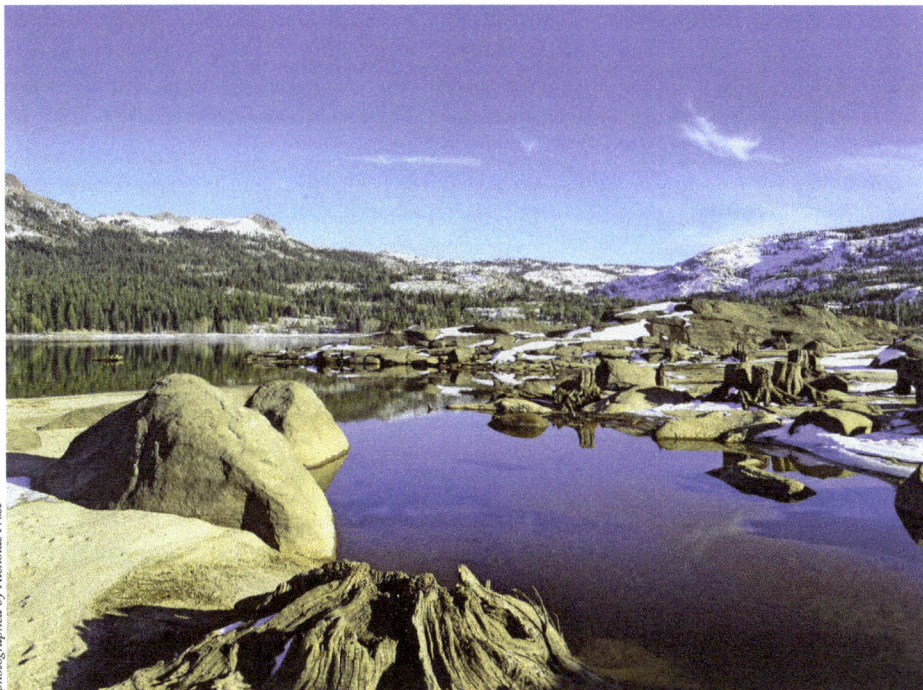

photographed by Nicholas Frost

KEY INFORMATION

LOCATION: CA 88, 52 miles east of Jackson, Kit Carson, CA 95666

OPERATED BY: Eldorado National Forest, Amador Ranger District

CONTACT: 209-295-4251; www.fs.usda.gov /eldorado

OPEN: June–October 15 (depending on road and weather conditions)

SITES: 61 total: 22 tent sites; 25 tent, trailer, or RV sites; 11 walk-in tent sites; 3 double tent sites

EACH SITE HAS: Picnic table, fireplace

ASSIGNMENT: 41 sites are reservable; 20 are first come, first served

REGISTRATION: At entrance; reserve at 877-444-6777 or recreation.gov

AMENITIES: Water, vault toilets; boat rental and campground store nearby at Kit Carson Lodge

PARKING: At individual site

FEE: $24, $5 extra vehicle

ELEVATION: 7,200'

RESTRICTIONS:

PETS: On leash only

FIRES: In fireplace

ALCOHOL: No restrictions

VEHICLES: No bicycles on trails; sites limited to 2 vehicles and 6 people

OTHER: Don't leave food out; 14-day stay limit

at the time—so fascinated, in fact, that it is rumored they would dig up the corpses of expired forty-niners to get their clothes and would often contract whatever disease had killed the unfortunate pilgrim.

If you come over the mountaintop from the west and look down at beautiful Silver Lake and the granite cliffs around it, you'll see that Silver Lake, like Caples Lake above it, is in a basin called a cirque. Cirques are formed when glaciers eat into the rock at its upper end. The ice slides down and takes the quarried rock with it, making room for more ice. Soon enough it digs out a basin. Usually, these basins or cirques appear in a series called paternosters—like Caples Lake and Silver Lake—so named because the lakes are in a string, like beads in a rosary.

Fishing Silver Lake is good fun, as the lake is not as heavily fished as nearby Lower Bear River Reservoir or Caples Lake. A car-top canoe or an inflatable is fine, as the lake is narrow and protected. There are also boats for rent at Silver Lake. Look for brook, brown, and rainbow trout. Most fishermen I saw headed for the northwest corner of the lake near the boat ramp, or they fished near Treasure Island, where the American River comes into the lake. Ask at the bait shop for what the fish were hitting the day before and where, and follow suit.

While some are fishing, others can go hiking. A great hike is up to Shealor Lake. It's about 3 miles round-trip and perfect for a day hike, incorporating lunch and a dip. Find the trailhead by driving 1.2 miles west of the turnoff for the Kit Carson Lodge (great cabins at the lodge if you're tired of the tent) from CA 88. There's a sign for Shealor Lake and a parking lot. Head up through the trees, and climb the granite slope to the top of the ridge. The gnarly-looking trees out in the wind are juniper and stunted lodgepole pines. Circle down through the rocks to the lake, and jump in. Where the rock cliffs fall away to ledges, the water warms up in the sun. The temperature is almost tenable for the non–polar bear.

Another good hike for lunch and a dip is up to Granite Lake. Drive past Kit Carson Lodge on the east side of the lake.

Call ahead before coming: the Carson Pass area is famous for snow. Indeed, on the first foray by the Mormon battalion, they ran into snow so deep a donkey fell into a drift and buried himself up to his ears. Fortunately, the men were able to grab the afflicted animal by his ears and drag him to safety. The Mormons held off their trip until July, when more of the snow had melted. Be sure to phone ahead, so you don't arrive and find the place snowed in.

If you reserve, mention that you are tent camping, because there are tent-only sites. These all seemed to be farther off the highway than the RV-capacity sites. Also, don't count on buying much more than ice and beer locally—bring everything else in from Jackson, down the hill.

Silver Lake East Campground

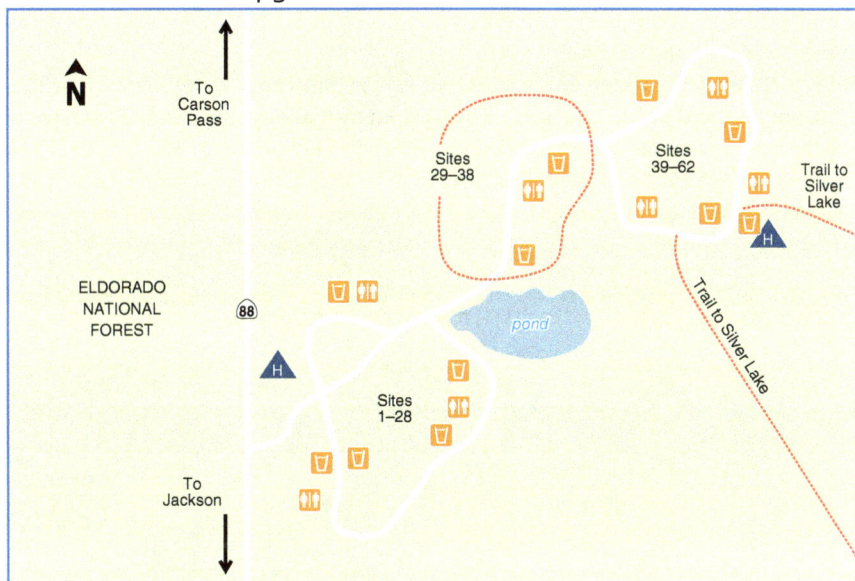

GETTING THERE

From Jackson, drive 52 miles east on CA 88 to the campground entrance on the right, past the Silver Lake dam.

GPS COORDINATES: N38° 40.324' W120° 7.160'

37

Woods Lake Campground

Beauty ★★★★★ / Privacy ★★★★★ / Spaciousness ★★★★★ / Quiet ★★★★ / Security ★★★★★ /
Cleanliness ★★★★★

Make an effort to camp here—the prettiest lake camping in the High Sierra.

Your first look at Woods Lake will make your head swim. This tiny blue gem is surrounded by mountains reaching to the sky. Waterfalls flash silver as they fall down from the melting snowfields. Boulders and islands along the water's edge glow warm and gray in the high-altitude sun. The needles are soft under the pines. A few anglers float around, fly-casting in their waders and inflatable devices. A family paddles by in a canoe (no motorboats allowed). Then you'll see the campground.

Woods Lake Campground is precious. Set up for tent campers, the first 14 or so sites have the fireplace and picnic table set well back from the parking space. You'll pitch your tent among the red penstemon–emblazoned rocks, down in a hollow, or up on a hillside. You have to come Sunday afternoon through Thursday to get a spot here. People come back year after year, and everyone you meet seems to have a story about camping here in summers past.

Round Top (10,381') is a prominent peak on the Carson Pass. Hikes to Winnemucca and Round Top Lakes, as well as Round Top Peak, are accessible from Woods Lake Campground.

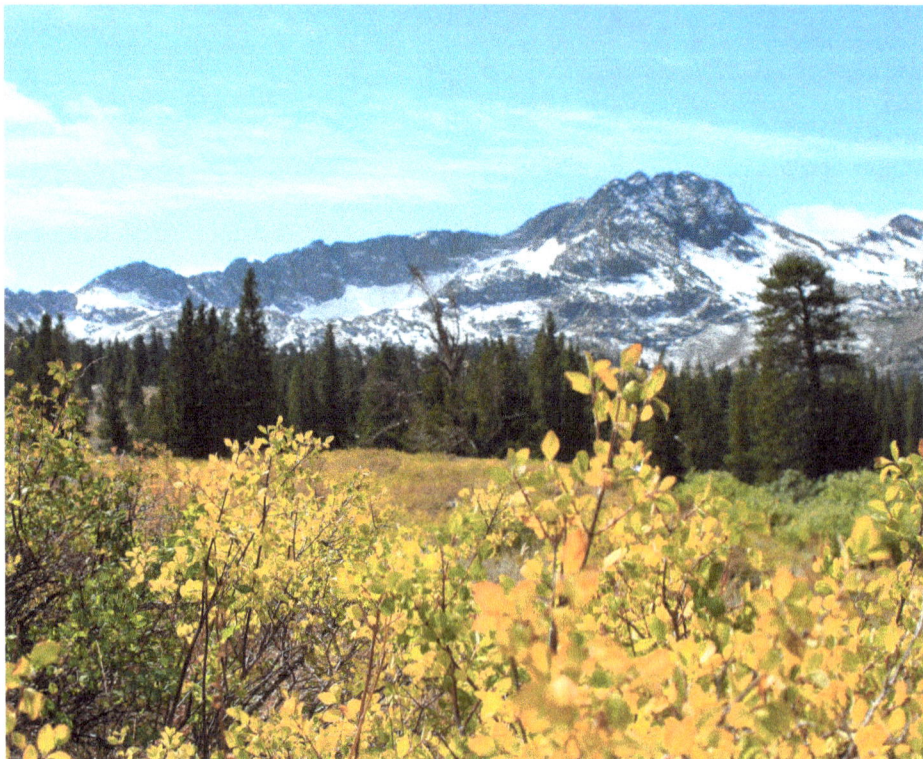

KEY INFORMATION

LOCATION: Woods Lake Road, 63.5 miles east of Jackson, Kirkwood, CA 95646

OPERATED BY: Eldorado National Forest, Amador Ranger District

CONTACT: 209-295-4251; www.fs.usda.gov /eldorado

OPEN: June 15–October 15 (weather permitting)

SITES: 23 single sites and 2 double sites for tents

EACH SITE HAS: Picnic table, fireplace

ASSIGNMENT: First come, first served; no reservations

REGISTRATION: At entrance

AMENITIES: Water, wheelchair-accessible vault toilets, picnic area; boat rental and campground store nearby at Caples Lake Resort

PARKING: At individual site

FEE: $24, $5 extra vehicle

ELEVATION: 8,200'

RESTRICTIONS:

PETS: On leash only

FIRES: In fireplace

ALCOHOL: No restrictions

VEHICLES: No RVs or trailers; maximum 2 vehicles and 6 people/single site; maximum 4 vehicles and 12 people/double site

OTHER: Don't leave food out; use bear boxes; 14-day stay limit

Good fun can be had just tramping around the lake, but be aware that you'll likely find some water to wade through along the way, as waterfalls run into the lake. There's also a swamp on the far side of the lake, which you can avoid by climbing up over the rocks and down the other side (though not without risk), but eventually the trail links back to the campground.

There are two trailheads near the campground. From either, you make a big arc through Winnemucca Lake and Round Top Lake, and back down to Woods Lake. The full trip is about 5 miles. Remember to watch the weather: it can snow here just about anytime. It's not a bad idea to pack one of those emergency rain parkas (sold in camping stores), along with a sweater, which could give you a margin of comfort if it does start storming.

Access one end of the trail from the day-use parking lot near Woods Lake. Cross the bridge over the stream and follow the signed trail to Winnemucca Lake. You'll walk first on the shoulder of a moraine (a ridge of rubble left by a retreating glacier), then into a pine forest. Spot the arrastra (a Mexican mining device for breaking up ore) on the right. Then the trail breaks out into a meadow filled with acres of wildflowers tumbling up toward the ridge and sky above. What an incredible sight! Only later, when we chatted with a nice woman hiking with a huge slobbering hound, did we learn that this wildflower spot is famous for its display.

Soon enough you'll come to Winnemucca Lake (named for a Paiute chief from Nevada), a sharp blue shard of water set in weathered gray granite. Two daring young hikers hastily breaststroked across to a warm boulder and flopped up on it like pink seals. Otherwise, there was just the sigh of the wind across the rocks and stunted pines.

A 4x4 signpost directs you to Round Top Lake. There's more huffing and puffing to this lake, and then the trail swings down around Lost Cabin Mine (posted against trespassers) and drops you at the campground near sites 14–16.

Fishing at Woods Lake and Winnemucca Lake is fine. I saw a few folks down at Woods Lake pull in some 10-inch rainbows at the Woods Creek end of the lake. But fishing here is not about what you catch, obviously. It is a religious experience, and most people seemed to approach it that way.

The little Carson Pass Information Center a few miles east on CA 88 is worth visiting—at least to see what books and pamphlets they have about the area. Read too the plaque outside about old Snowshoe Thompson. This old boy was tough as nails and makes our ironworkers of today look like a bunch of wimps.

Remember to bring supplies. Caples Lake Resort has a tiny store that sells ice, beer, and fishing gear but not much else. The nearest real grocery store is across the pass at Woodfords. For campers who strike out at Woods Lake, I suggest going over the pass to the Blue Lakes.

Woods Lake Campground

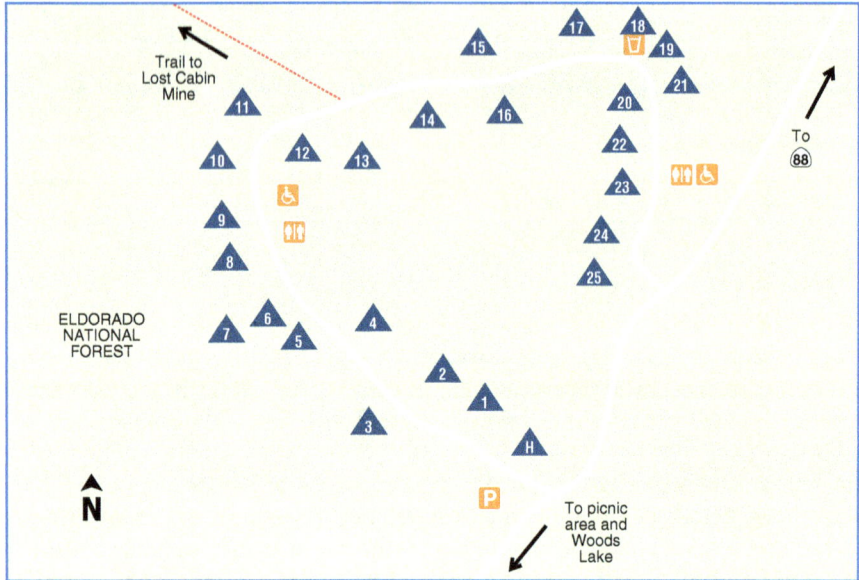

GETTING THERE

From Jackson, drive east about 60 miles on CA 88, past Caples Lake, to the turnoff to Woods Lake Campground on the right. Go about 2 miles. The campground entrance is on the right before you reach Woods Lake.

GPS COORDINATES: N38° 41.255' W120° 0.562'

38

Grover Hot Springs State Park Campgrounds

Beauty ★★★★ / Privacy ★★★ / Spaciousness ★★★★ / Quiet ★★★ / Security ★★★★★ /
Cleanliness ★★★★

Great for kids in the summer; good adult camping the rest of the year

First off—Quaking Aspen Campground and Toiyabe Campground are just different loops in one campground in Grover Hot Springs State Park. Secondly, it is a family park. If you're looking for peace and quiet, you don't want to be here in the summer when school's out—the place is full of kids.

But if you have kids, Grover Hot Springs (named after Alvin M. Grover, one of the original Anglo owners) is the place to be. There are lots of other kids to play with yours, so you can kick back for a change. There's a nice warm swimming pool watched over by healthy, young lifeguards; a stream full of fish and other interesting denizens; miles of trails up rounded hills; miles of nontrafficked roads to bike on; grassy meadows; a nearby Western town with a museum, supplies, and horse rentals; a nature trail; hot showers; flush toilets; and a big, uncrowded camp to run around in like a wild animal.

The corollary to all the summer activity is that you must reserve, reserve, reserve. Make sure you have a campsite before dragging your kids all the way up here to find the place

The Scossa cabin, circa 1935, stands next to the hot pool at Grover Hot Springs State Park Campground. The pools are fed by natural hot springs and are open year-round.

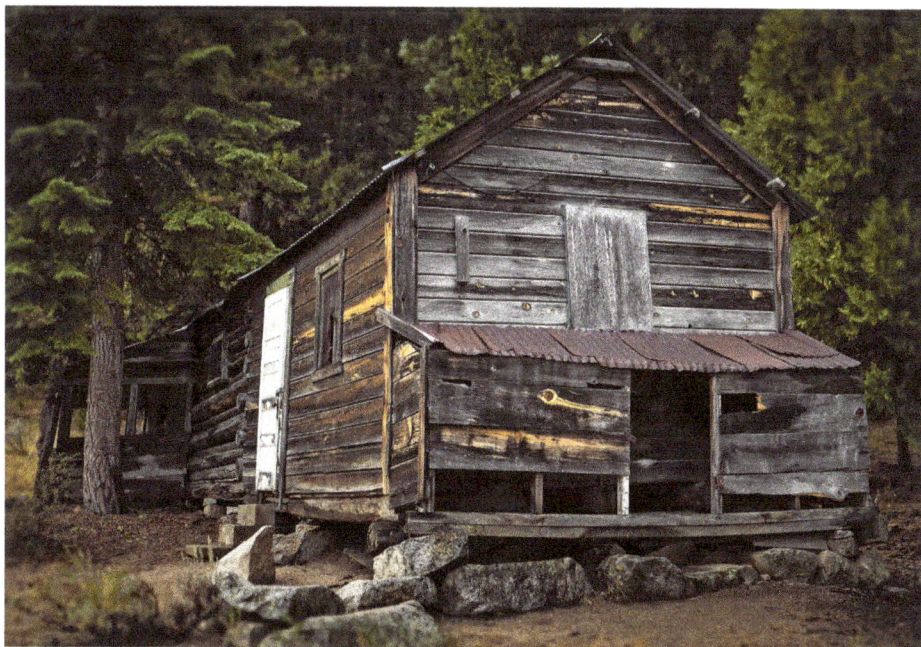

KEY INFORMATION

LOCATION: 3415 Hot Springs Road, Markleeville, CA 96120

OPERATED BY: Grover Hot Springs State Park

CONTACT: 530-694-2248, www.parks.ca.gov

OPEN: Year-round

SITES: 24 tent sites; 45 sites for tents, RVs, or trailers; 2 wheelchair-accessible sites

EACH SITE HAS: Picnic table, fireplace, food locker, water faucet every 3 sites

ASSIGNMENT: First come, first served; reservations recommended

REGISTRATION: By entrance; reserve at 800-444-7275 or reservecalifornia.com

AMENITIES: Water, flush toilets, showers (except in the winter), wood for sale

PARKING: At individual site

FEE: $35, $25 off-season, $8 nonrefundable reservation fee

ELEVATION: 6,000'

RESTRICTIONS:

PETS: On leash only

FIRES: In fireplace

ALCOHOL: No restrictions

VEHICLES: Trailers up to 24 feet, RVs up to 27 feet

OTHER: Reservations recommended on holidays and in summer; hot springs pool normally closed 2 to 3 weeks in September for annual maintenance, generally right after Labor Day; keep food in lockers

jammed. Some of the campsites here are by Hot Springs Creek. At first that might seem enviable, but this is where the fishermen fish and the excited kids play in the stream. Better to reserve a site off the creek, backed into the woods. Stay away from the bathrooms as well.

During the rest of the year, Grover Hot Springs is wide open for killjoy geezers who don't thrill to the trill of youthful voices. This is a beautiful park. It's well run and clean. The hike up to the waterfall is just enough to get the blood pumping without stressing the pacemaker. The hot springs bath adjacent to the pool is guaranteed rejuvenation with lingering powers, and somehow, the waters issue forth from the earth without that rotten-egg sulfur smell. When the Sierra Nevada rose as one huge chunk millions of years ago, the violent changes caused faulting—that is, cracks in the massive rock structure. Water from the surface, then, works its way down through the faults to the magma where the rock is hot as hell, then boils back to the surface as hot spring waters replete with minerals it has dissolved along its way. The minerals include sodium chloride; sodium sulfate; sodium carbonate; calcium carbonate; magnesium carbonate; and a little iron, alumina, and silica. This means lots of salt. I definitely felt better after my cure. The water is hot, about 103°F, which is cooler than the 148°F that it was when it left the ground. The hot pool is right next to the swimming pool.

There are good hikes around the camp. Find campsites 35 and 36, and you'll be at the extra-vehicle parking lot, where a marked trail heads west for the waterfall. It heads along beautiful meadows and through pine woods—mostly Jeffrey pines. Sniff the bark: the Jeffrey pine smells just like vanilla. Another salient fact that I learned from the Grover Hot Springs State Park Guide to the Park's Transition Walk concerns the Jeffrey pine's cones, which are a primary food source for the reddish-black Douglas squirrel. The guide asserts that "of the millions of seeds produced during the lifetime of a pine tree, only one, on the average, will grow into a new tree!"

On the trail to the falls, you'll cross some small springs and soon enough hear the falls. When the water is low, you can go up beside the streambed to the falls. In spring, however, count on climbing up the rocks just ahead of you to approach the falls. The round-trip should take you a little more than an hour.

Nearby Markleeville, population 210, is worth a trip. Visit the museum at the Alpine County Historical Complex. In 1861 Bactrian camels from Mongolia were brought here to be used as pack animals. Bad move. Conditions in the Gobi desert are a lot different from those in the Sierra Nevada. However, modern packers have made good use of the Peruvian llama, obviously better bred for life in these parts.

Another fun cultural trip is to Genoa for the Mormon Station Historical State Monument. This little park, with its stockade, museum, and picnic facilities, used to be a relief station for traveling pioneers. Basically, the tired travelers staggered into the station and were promptly overcharged for their bed, bath, and meal. Most men arrived on horseback and left on foot. The owners of the station fattened up the horses and sold them back to new travelers for more cash. Right across the street stands the oldest tavern in Nevada, where the fleeced traveler could go to drown his sorrows.

Grover Hot Springs State Park Campgrounds

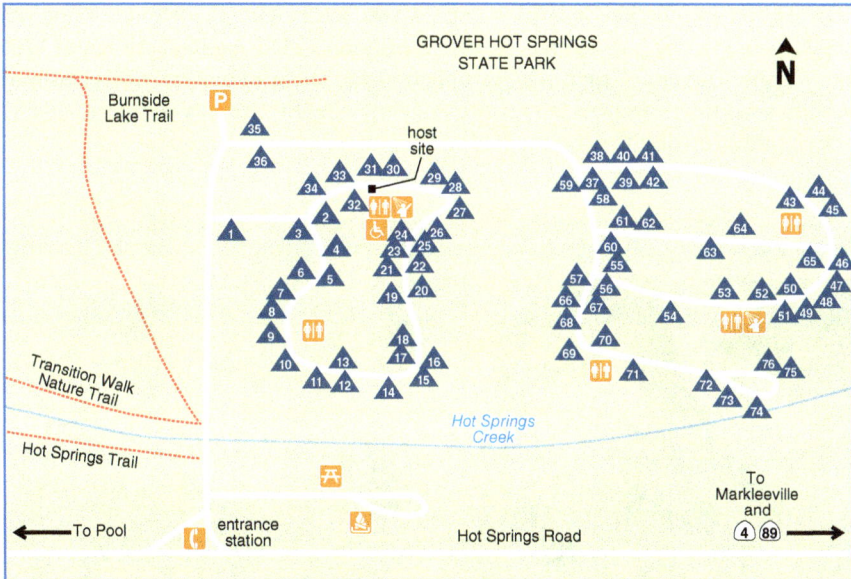

GETTING THERE

From Markleeville, head about 4 miles west on Hot Springs Road.

GPS COORDINATES: N38° 41.977' W119° 50.150'

39

Wrights Lake Campground

Beauty ★★★★★ / Privacy ★★★ / Spaciousness ★★★ / Quiet ★★★ / Security ★★★ / Cleanliness ★★★

Reserve ahead—this is the best place to bring kids. It is stunningly beautiful, too.

Reserve your site six months ahead. Bring the kids because Wrights Lake Campground is perfect for kids of all ages. The lake is clean and warm, ideal for swimming off the rocks and shore, or from canoes and small inflatables on the water. This is a made-to-order movie set for a coming-of-age film. The campground is small and intimate. For once the tent-only sites get the best real estate—down by the lake—while the RVers are off on the other side of the dam. The sites are private, with boulders and coppices of pines blocking them from one another. The plateau area that Wrights Lake occupies is sylvan and warm, with crisscrossing streams—more meadow than the harsher oceans of granite farther south toward Yosemite.

This place is popular—everybody has a smile on their face. Folks from Sacramento and San Francisco plan a year ahead to spend their vacations here. All you can hear is the sound of birds singing and the kids splashing in the water and laughing. Even the campground's namesake was a happy guy. Friends on an expedition in 1881 wrote about James William Albert Wright: "Captain Wright was the only fleshy member of our party. His ribs were so encased in such thick layers of fatty tissue that, knowing his inability to freeze, we elected that he should sleep on the windward side of the camp."

Placid Wright's Lake (motorboats prohibited) is an excellent place to bring the kayak, stand-up paddleboard or canoe.

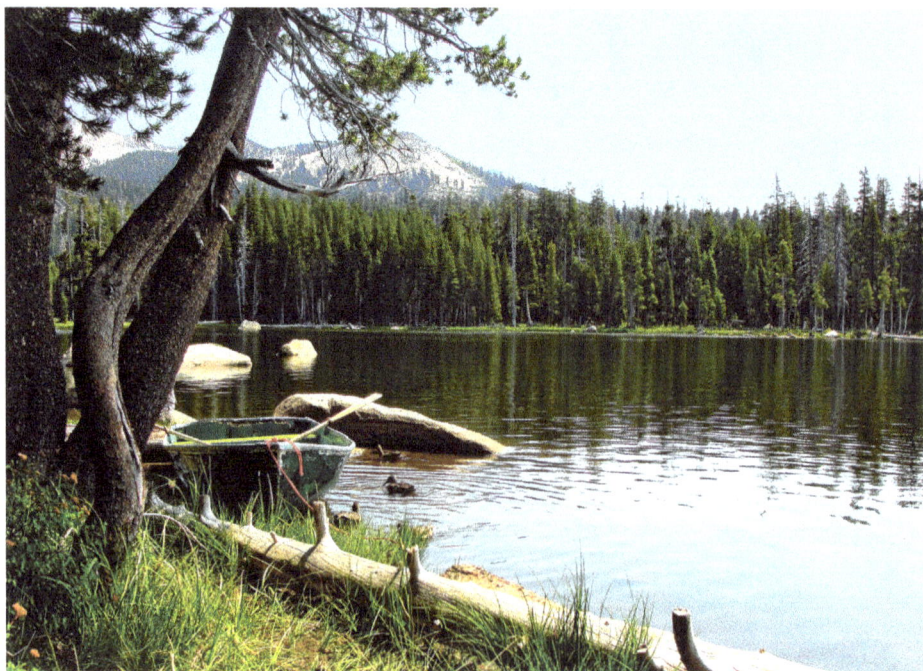

photographed by Rick Kasper

KEY INFORMATION

LOCATION: Wrights Lake Road, 43 miles east of Placerville on US 50, Kyburz, CA 95720

OPERATED BY: Eldorado National Forest, Pacific Ranger District

INFORMATION: 530-644-2349; www.fs.usda.gov/eldorado

OPEN: Late June–mid-October (depending on road and weather conditions)

SITES: 67 total: 33 tent sites, 24 tent or RV sites, 3 double sites, 9 walk-in tent sites

EACH SITE HAS: Picnic table, fire ring, food locker

ASSIGNMENT: First come, first served; reservations required and available July 5–Labor Day

REGISTRATION: At entrance; reserve at 877-444-6777 or recreation.gov

AMENITIES: Water (may be shut off after Labor Day), vault toilets, wheelchair-accessible sites

PARKING: At individual site

FEE: $20, $36 for double site, $5 extra vehicle, $9 nonrefundable reservation fee

ELEVATION: 7,000'

RESTRICTIONS:

PETS: On leash only

FIRES: In fire ring

ALCOHOL: No restrictions

VEHICLES: RVs up to 50 feet; motorboats prohibited; maximum of 2 vehicles and 6 people/site for single sites; maximum 2 vehicles and 12 people per site for double sites

OTHER: Don't leave food out; 14-day stay limit

You have to bring some kind of flotation device along. Motorboats are not allowed, so midnight paddles are a widespread Wrights Lake practice. Light car-top canoes or kayaks are best adapted to the lake, but any inflatable will do. Buy an electric pump to plug into your car's cigarette lighter and a repair kit. These inflatables are fun on high mountain lakes. They get you out of the freezing water, off the shore, and into the sun.

Wrights Lake is accessed from US 50, which was built as a toll road by Colonel John Calhoun "Cock-Eye" Johnson. He made a ton of money on wagons heading for Virginia City, Nevada (well worth a visit—go on a weekday). Cock-Eye's toll road was rumored to be "five-feet-deep by a hundred-and-thirty-miles long, and composed mostly of mountains, snow, and mud." Now cars and buses (gambler's specials) fly up and down this road. It's kind of unnerving, and you'll need to watch carefully for Wrights Lake Road, which comes abruptly on a curve, so be mindful of the frantic traffic.

Bring lots of ice and supplies. The nearest reliable gasoline, ice, and groceries are in Meyers to the east over Echo Summit and Riverton to the west. Bring an extra cooler packed with ice and duct-taped shut. Put a wet blanket on it to cool it by evaporation. Put drinks in a little six-pack cooler so folks won't be opening and closing the food cooler all day long. Make a menu and stick to it—it's amazing how little food you need if it is planned out. Don't count on "living off the lake," although people do catch rainbow and brown trout—the lake is stocked, and some of the brown trout that survive through the winter get to be pretty big.

Hiking around Wrights Lake is fun. Many of the other day hikes require permits, which you can conveniently get at the campground. The last time I was up there, we hiked up to Smith Lake. The hike is a killer but has the asset of leaving from the campground. Just hike up the road on the east side of Wrights Lake to the Twin and Grouse Lakes Trailhead. Cross the fence and walk up through the meadow. At the beginning of July it was packed with flowers.

After maybe 0.5 mile, the trail splits. Go right up the slope; the trail climbs. Pass a sign for the Desolation Wilderness, and go right when the trail splits. When you reach a trail signed for Twin/Island Lakes, go right again. This climb is a bear until you get to Grouse Lake. If you have any sand left in you, go left around the shore and follow the trail through the swamp, up to Hemlock Lake.

Keep going to the right of Hemlock Lake and stagger on up the mountain to Smith Lake. This lake is good dipping, and you're going to need it. You've only walked 4 miles from the campground, but 3 of them have been straight up. Imagine how you'd feel if you were carrying a 50-pound pack. No wonder John Muir went hiking in his greatcoat with all his provisions in his pockets.

Wrights Lake Campground

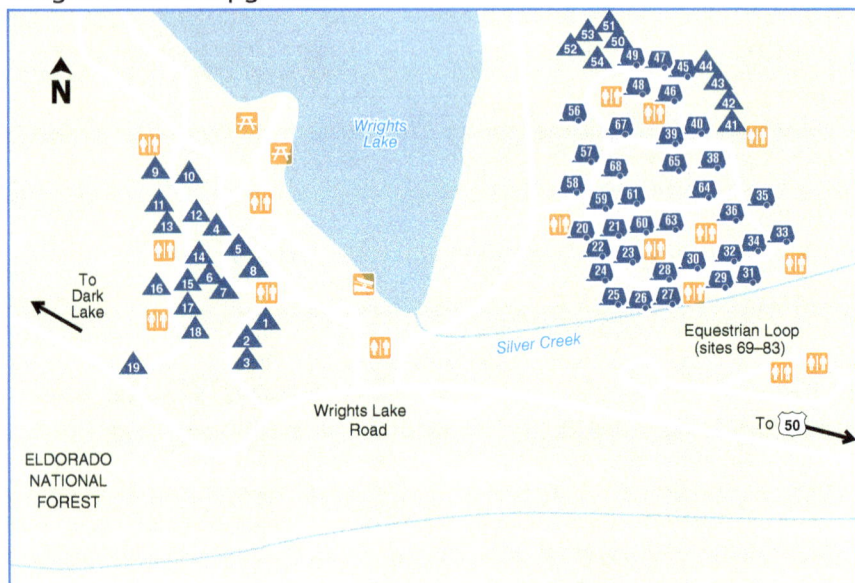

GETTING THERE

From Placerville, drive 34 miles east on US 50. Turn left on Wrights Lake Road (watch the turn—it's dangerous), and go 8 miles up the narrow road to the campground.

GPS COORDINATES: N38° 50.677' W120° 14.207'

40

D. L. Bliss State Park Campgrounds

Beauty ★★★★★ / Privacy ★★★ / Spaciousness ★★★★ / Quiet ★★★ / Security ★★★★★ / Cleanliness ★★★★★

Come armed with reservations, kids, water gear, a camera, and hiking boots—this is high-profile California camping.

Lake Tahoe, the queen of California lakes, faces a mountain of woes—population and pollution threaten the lake's natural beauty. But if you come to D. L. Bliss State Park and hike down the Rubicon Trail toward Emerald Bay State Park, you'll see Tahoe almost as Mark Twain did. He wrote, "The air up there is very pure and fine, bracing and delicious. It is the same air the angels breathe. . . . The view was always fascinating, bewitching, entrancing." Tahoe still has the same effect, and D. L. Bliss State Park shows her off at her best.

Who was D. L. Bliss? Finding the answer took a bit of research. Finally, I tracked down Mr. Duane LeRoy Bliss. No nature lover, he was actually a ruthless lumberman who made a fortune cutting down most of the trees in the Tahoe Basin. After his demise, an heir guiltily donated some of the denuded acres to the State of California.

Now, besides being reforested and magically beautiful, D. L. Bliss State Park is a parent's delight. The place is crawling with kids playing under the pines and climbing the rounded

Camp on the shores of Lake Tahoe, the largest alpine lake in North America, and enjoy the cool, clear waters, as well as a host of watersports, hiking, and biking nearby.

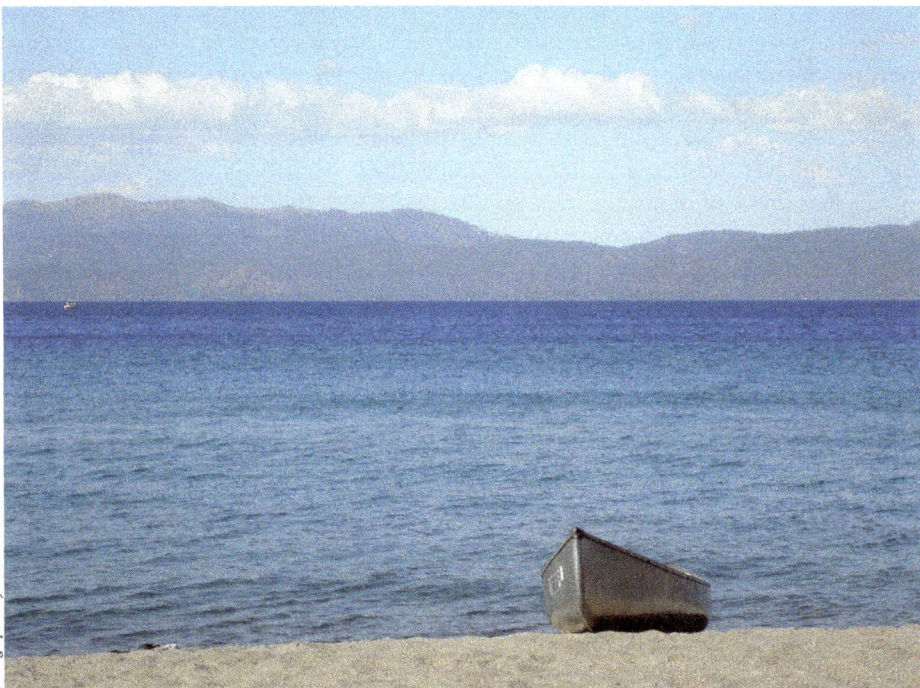

photographed by Martha Riecks

KEY INFORMATION

LOCATION: 9881 CA 89, South Lake Tahoe, CA 96150

OPERATED BY: D. L. Bliss State Park

CONTACT: 530-525-7277; www.parks.ca.gov

OPEN: May–September

SITES: 168 sites for tents or RVs under 16 feet

EACH SITE HAS: Picnic table, fireplace, food locker

ASSIGNMENT: First come, first served; reservations recommended

REGISTRATION: 1 mile past entrance; reserve at 800-444-7275 or reservecalifornia.com

AMENITIES: Water, flush toilets, showers, wood for sale

PARKING: At individual site

FEE: $45 for lakeshore sites, $35 for others, $8 nonrefundable reservation fee

ELEVATION: 6,920'

RESTRICTIONS:

PETS: Allowed only on leash in park; dogs not allowed on trails, beaches, or Vikingsholm area

FIRES: In fireplace

ALCOHOL: No restrictions

VEHICLES: RVs up to 15 feet for trailers and 18 feet for motor homes

OTHER: Reservations required on holidays and summer weekends; 8-person maximum; keep food and toiletries in lockers provided (required by law)

boulders in the campground. We brought our big-city niece to Bliss, and within moments she was running around the campground playing hide-and-seek with all the kids. The flush toilets are immaculately clean, and the hot showers are heavenly after a day of swimming down at Lester Beach (the best beach in Tahoe for kids) and hiking the Rubicon Trail to Emerald Bay and back.

There are three campground areas. One area, campsites 141–168, is close to Lester Beach. These sites must be reserved. You must specifically request them, and they cost $10 more per night than the rest of the campsites. The sites are packed in—tents only—and a little sandy, so it's not a bad idea to bring a tarp or strip of Astroturf to put in front of your tent or, better still, a basin to fill with water so the kiddies can dip their feet before dragging sand into the tent and ultimately into your sleeping bag.

The next group of campsites, sites 91–140, are 0.5 mile from Lester Beach. These sites are more spread out but still heavily used. I like camping still farther up the hill at sites 1–90 (site 22 is great!), where it is roomier and the ground is covered with a bed of pine needles. You're a mile from the beach here, but you can easily walk or drive down (folks camping can always park below even if the day-use parking lot is full). This is kid-o-rama as well and has the advantage of not being on the main drag.

On the beach, the sand is white and clean and perfect for making sand castles. This is good news, as the water is freezing and fit only for walruses or Nordic rites of manhood. A couple of handy items here are one of those cheap little blow-up boats and an electric pump that plugs into the car's cigarette lighter. With this outfit, you can float around the buoyed-off swimming area and read a novel. Or the kids can splash in and out of it and dump each other into the gelid water. There are no lifeguards, but people keep a pretty close eye on their kids and everyone else's.

Fishing at Lake Tahoe is either really great (when you score) or a total shutout. The clear, beautiful water is the problem. Fish need algae to support a food chain. Still, mackinaw trout, rainbow trout, and kokanee salmon can be found. They tend to stay at low depths in areas that provide them some cover—find mackinaws near Emerald Bay, in the northwest, and off the south shore. Rainbows lurk anywhere there's a rocky bottom. Nobody seemed to know where kokanees hide. They just show up, and if you happen to be there—eureka! Everyone agrees the fishing is best in the early morning and evening and on cloudy days.

The biking in D. L. Bliss State Park is poor because the park is on a fairly steep hill. Still, there is good biking around Lake Tahoe. One paved bike path leads to the Truckee River, a good ways down the northeast shore of the lake. Another begins below Emerald Bay State Park and curls around the south shore.

Hiking the Rubicon Trail is a must. You can access the trail (stop at the visitor center for a map) just south of Lester Beach or from a parking area just below the check-in station. Just cross the road and you'll see the sign for the trail.

Avoid Lake Tahoe's southeast corner unless you can bear 8 miles of motels and restaurants with outdoorsy-sounding names. CA 89 from the north or south is much friendlier. Shop in Tahoe City near the north end of the lake. A little store at Meeks Bay offers ice, beer, and sundries.

D.L. Bliss State Park Campgrounds

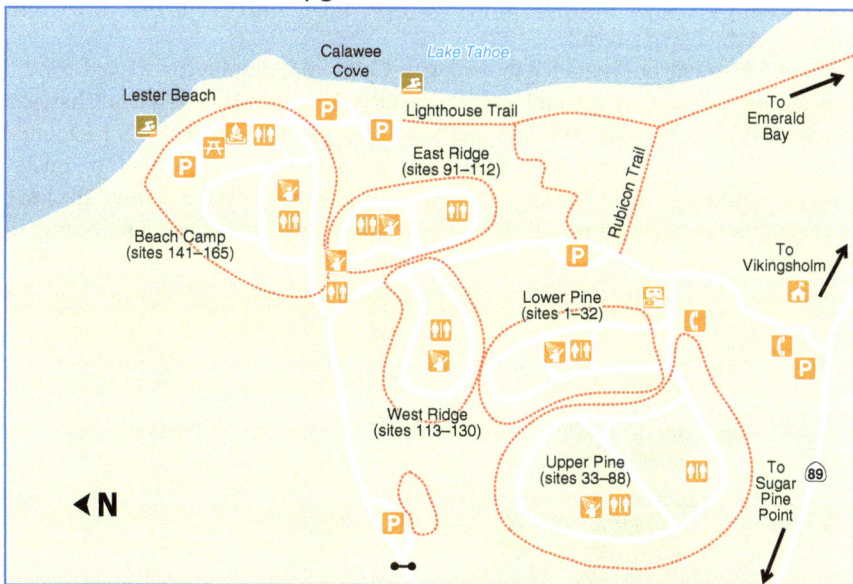

GETTING THERE

From the intersection of CA 89 and US 50 in South Lake Tahoe, drive 11 miles north on CA 89 past the entrance to Emerald Bay State Park, to the D. L. Bliss State Park entrance on the right. Meeks Bay is a few miles north of the park entrance.

GPS COORDINATES: N38° 58.944' W120° 6.085'

41

Sardine Lake and Salmon Creek Campgrounds

Beauty ★★★★★ / Privacy ★★★★ / Spaciousness ★★★★★ / Quiet ★★★★ / Security ★★★ / Cleanliness ★★★

These twin campgrounds are base camps for endless Sierra Nevada adventure.

Wonderful Salmon Creek trills past the Salmon Creek Campground, and Sardine Lake Campground is a mile away, just below the Sardine Lakes. Nestled into the still-pristine Gold Lakes area, these campgrounds have it all: excellent fishing and hiking, fabulous scenery, and epic mountain biking.

Scooped out of the flank of Sierra Buttes (8,587'), Lower and Upper Sardine Lakes are classic glacier tarns caused by the carving and scouring action of a glacier as it passed over bedrock. The low spots filled with water and became tarns. How beautiful! The Sardine Lakes are blue and clear and mirror the snow and rocks in the Sierra Buttes above. (Read the chapter titled "The Glacier Lakes" in John Muir's *The Mountains of California* for a rhapsodic description of the life of a tarn.)

No wonder the forty-niners fell in love with California, despite the wicked hand Lady Luck dealt them. Still, they remembered the beauty of California, and when Charles Nordoff (author of *California for Travelers and Settlers*) came through in 1872, he found that many of the forty-niners had stayed or returned to Gold Country to live out their days.

Every site at Sardine Lake Campground has a full view of the Sierra Buttes. The last time I was there, they were brushing out the campground, so we moved half a mile away to the

Mills Peak Fire Lookout is a great place to begin the delightful 9-mile, 3,167-foot downhill mountain bike descent over swooping singletrack trail to the intersection of CA 89 and Gold Lakes Highway.

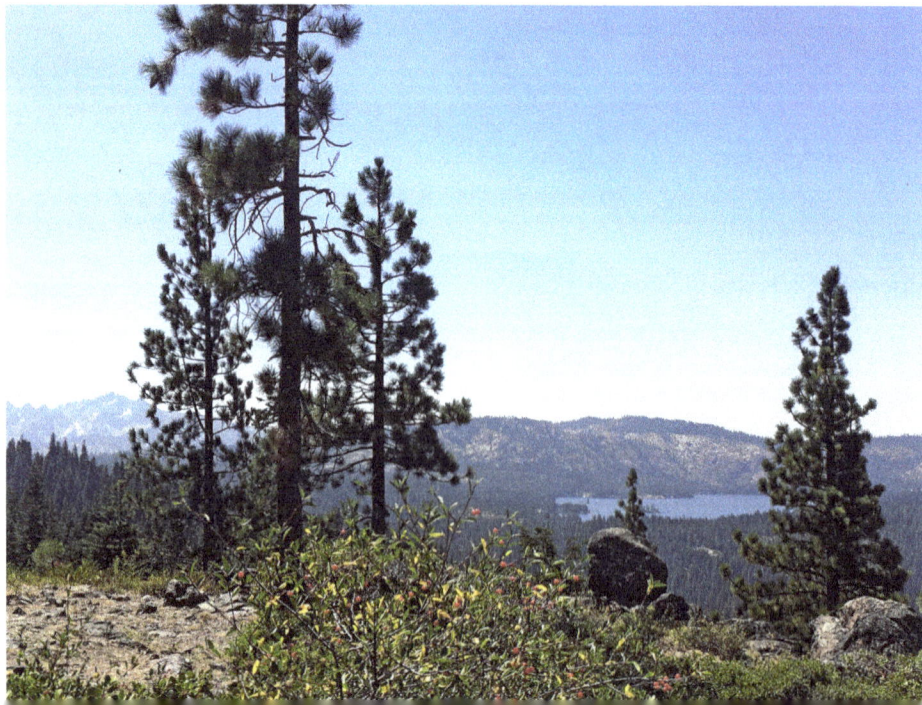

KEY INFORMATION

LOCATION: Gold Lake Highway, 2 miles north of Bassetts, Calpine, CA 96124

OPERATED BY: Tahoe National Forest, Yuba River Ranger District

CONTACT: 530-478-6253; www.fs.usda.gov /tahoe

OPEN: June–October (depending on road and weather conditions)

SITES: Sardine Lake: 29 total, 15 sites for trailers; Salmon Creek: 31 total, 7 sites for trailers

EACH SITE HAS: Picnic table, fireplace

ASSIGNMENT: Reserve at 877-444-677 or recreation.gov

REGISTRATION: At entrance

AMENITIES: Water, vault toilets

PARKING: At individual site

FEE: $24, $5 extra vehicle

ELEVATION: 5,800'

RESTRICTIONS:

PETS: On leash only

FIRES: In fireplace

ALCOHOL: No restrictions

VEHICLES: RVs and small trailers allowed (no hookups)

OTHER: Don't leave food out

Salmon Creek Campground, where our site backed up to the creek. Many of the sites there offer views of the mountains, but the rushing waters of Salmon Creek are equally scenic. The only slight catch in this otherwise fantastic campground is the road on the hill above the campground. From time to time, the muffler on a lumber truck overwhelms the splash of the creek, but this is a national forest, land of many uses.

A few hundred yards up toward Sardine Lake is Sand Pond, which offers good swimming. It is round, a couple hundred yards across, and shallow enough for the light-sand bottom to pick up the sun. In early June, Sand Pond is warm enough to sit in the water in an aluminum chair with a book. Formed by a mining operation of the nearby All American Gold Mine, Sand Pond is prime for aquatic kids.

Early in the morning, Sardine Lake is besieged with anglers who troll slowly across the water (the speed limit is 5 miles per hour) before disappointment or triumph brings them in for lunch. Some of them stay in the neat cabins at the foot of the lake. I'm told the food in the lodge there is spectacular. I eyeballed the menu in the window, and it looked decidedly haute cuisine. We met an older gent fishing nearby, who told us he rents a cabin every summer on Sardine Lake.

He told us about the hummingbirds, too. It seems there are seven species in Northern California, and six of them breed around Sardine Lake. I've actually seen and identified five: rufous, calliope, Anna's, broad-tailed, and black-chinned. They come iridescent green, blue, and red, beating their wings about 75 times per second, with their hearts pumping 500 times a minute. They are so quick and small you need binoculars to really take a measure of them. The prettiest is the smallest: the calliope, with exotic reddish throat whiskers. This little bird strengthens its nest with spider silk.

There is so much to do in this area it's astounding. Fat-tire adventure seekers won't want to miss the world-renowned Downieville Downhill mountain bike ride. This classic section, for strong intermediate and advanced riders, features 14 miles of tight and technical singletrack trail that drops almost 5,000 feet into the cute, Old West gold-mining town of Downieville.

Either set up a shuttle within your group (the trailhead is less than 5 miles from the campground, but you'll also need pickup in Downieville post-ride) or book a shuttle with Downieville mountain bike outfitter Yuba Expeditions (yubaexpeditions.com). To find the trailhead from the campground, head out Sardine Lake Road toward Gold Lake Highway, and make a hairpin left on Packer Lake Road. Follow it 4 miles to Packer Saddle, and begin on the Butcher Trail. For specific trail details, consult mtbproject.com.

Another good, slightly less technical ride can be found just a short jaunt up Gold Lake Highway at the Mill Peak Fire Lookout. It's a 9-mile, 3,167-foot descent that starts from the top and finishes at the intersection of Gold Lake Highway and CA 89.

For the less inclined to descend, good, peaceful fun can be had right at the campground. Take a hike on the Sand Pond Interpretive Trail from the campground. Bring a picnic lunch to the Frazier Falls overlook. And check out the sunset from Upper Sardine Lake. You really can't go wrong in this kind of paradise.

Sardine Lake and Salmon Creek Campgrounds

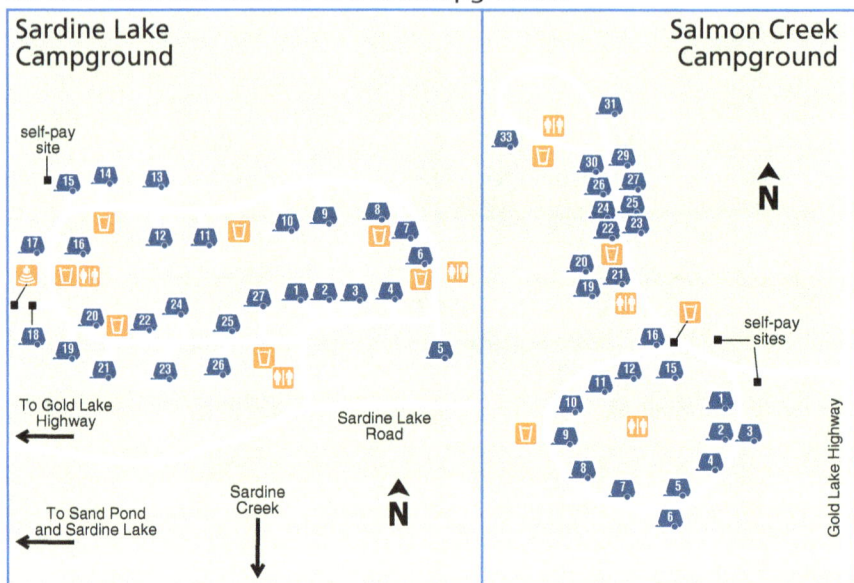

GETTING THERE

From Sierra City, go north on CA 49 about 5 miles to the junction with Gold Lake Highway. Go a little over a mile north to the entrance to Sardine Lake Campground on your left. For Salmon Creek Campground, stay on Gold Lake Highway a few hundred yards more to the entrance on your left.

GPS COORDINATES: N39° 37.127' W120° 37.046'

42

⛺ Wyandotte Campground

Beauty ★★★★ / Privacy ★★★★★ / Spaciousness ★★★★★ / Quiet ★★★★★ / Security ★★★★★ /
Cleanliness ★★★★★

Bring your fishing pole, bathing suit, and anything that floats.

First off, note that Little Grass Valley Reservoir is not in the outskirts of the gold country town of Grass Valley. It's not even in the same county. Little Grass Valley Reservoir, a 1,615-acre man-made lake nestled in the mountains of Plumas County, collects water from the Feather River watershed. Wyandotte is one of six campgrounds around the reservoir. Sites at Red Feather, Running Deer, and Horse Camp are reservable, while Wyandotte, Peninsula Tent, and Black Rock are not. Peninsula Tent is a good option if Wyandotte is full; Peninsula Tent has forested walk-in sites a short distance from the lake, but it sits right off the lake access road and can be a bit noisy. Wyandotte is more scenic and peaceful.

The sites at Wyandotte are situated along a straight road, with two tiny loops at either end. The campground slopes uphill from the shoreline, with sites at the lower end (21–29) offering the closest lake access, via a short path, to one of the reservoir's boat ramps and the shoreline. Some of the sites in the upper part of the campground offer partial views to the reservoir. The campground is shaded by a thick forest of tall ponderosa pine, sugar pine, and white fir, with little understory vegetation. To compensate for the lack of screening, most of the sites are very well spaced.

Recreational opportunities abound on Little Grass Valley Reservoir, with six campgrounds along its shores.

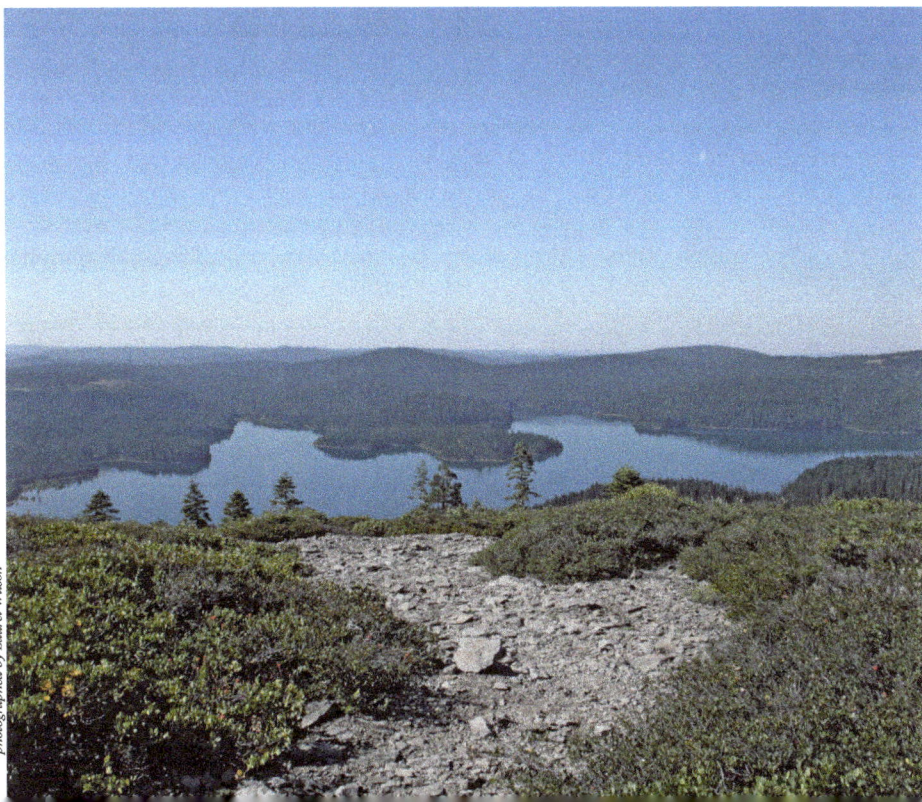

photographed by Laurel Wilson

KEY INFORMATION

LOCATION: Peninsula Road, 5 miles from La Porte, Little Grass Valley, CA 96053

OPERATED BY: Plumas National Forest, Feather River Ranger District

CONTACT: 530-534-6500; www.fs.usda.gov/plumas

OPEN: Memorial Day–October

SITES: 26 single sites for tents or RVs up to 50 feet, 2 double sites

EACH SITE HAS: Picnic table and fire ring

ASSIGNMENT: First come, first served; reservations available

REGISTRATION: Self-register at information area in middle of campground; 12 sites reservable at 877-444-6777 or recreation.gov

AMENITIES: Flush toilets, drinking water (sometimes unavailable, so call ahead or bring your own to be safe)

PARKING: At individual site

FEE: $23 single, $38 double

ELEVATION: 5,100'

RESTRICTIONS:

PETS: On leash

FIRES: In established pits or rings only

ALCOHOL: No restrictions

VEHICLES: 6 people and 2 vehicles/site maximum

OTHER: 14-day stay limit

Lots of pine needles form soft pads for tent pitches, but when walking barefoot, watch out for the small, sharp-tipped ponderosa pine cones strewn on the ground, and when setting up your tent or comfy chair, beware of the sugar pine cones falling from above—these cones range from 10 to 24 inches in length, and when one falls nearby you'll sit up and take notice. (If one falls on your tent while you're napping . . . well, it's better not to ponder this—be proactive.) Some of the sites facing the reservoir are a bit sloped, but each seems to have enough level ground for at least one tent.

Wyandotte opens around Memorial Day, before the other larger campgrounds around the lake, and when we camped here in early June, there were still some patches of snow off the sides of Little Grass Valley Road, although the day and night temperatures were wonderfully mild. From the rocky shoreline we plunged into the water, which was cold but warm enough for a short swim—it was so early in the season, the air was barely hot enough to encourage a longer dip. When we saw boats floating placidly along the lake, we wished for a canoe. Fishing is popular, with the reservoir supporting rainbow trout, German brown, and kokanee salmon. The roar of powerboats is occasionally audible from the campground but competes well with the sound of the wind through the trees.

You can hike on a path around the reservoir (it's 13.5 miles all the way around), but for a more scenic hike, you can drive to two nearby trailheads: trek part of the Pacific Crest Trail from the Fowler Peak trailhead, or hike the Hartman Bar Trail to the Middle Fork of the Feather River. Pick up the Plumas National Forest map from an outdoor retailer to find your way there.

We enjoyed excellent bird-watching right in our campground, observing western tanagers (males are particularly conspicuous yellow-breasted, red-headed birds) in the surrounding trees, and a trio of ospreys (fish hawks) soaring and calling overhead all day long. At night, owls hooted back and forth, and in the morning we rose to coyote howls in the distance.

Once you leave Oroville, the trip to Little Grass Valley Reservoir passes through a series of small towns and settlements, with very few services. La Porte is small and offers limited facilities, most notably a restaurant and tiny general store. Your best bet to stock up on supplies is Oroville, where you can gas up and purchase food and firewood. In La Porte there was no wood for sale in the store, but the town hosts a quirky firewood barren of sorts—follow the signs to buy a few armfuls of wood for your campfire.

Wyandotte Campground

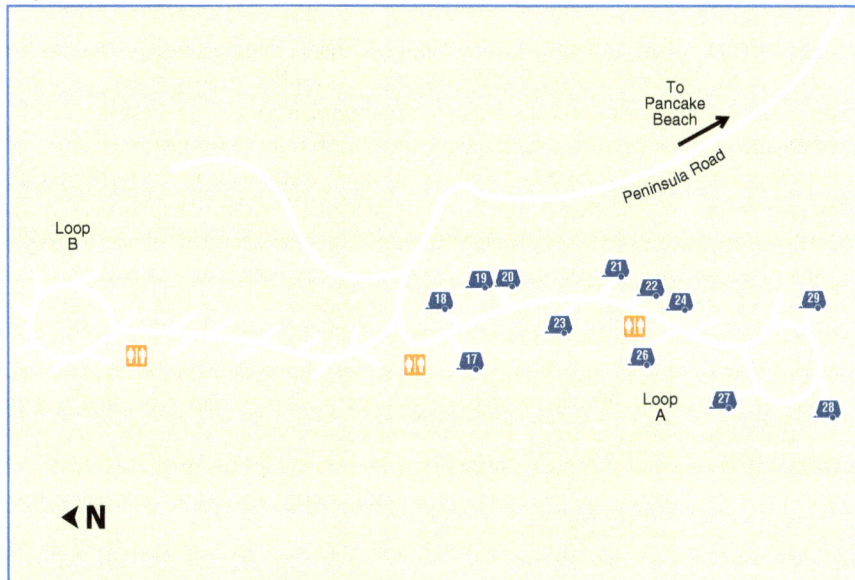

To
Pancake
Beach

Peninsula Road

Loop
B

Loop
A

19 20 21 22 24 18 23 26 17 27 28 29

◄ N

GETTING THERE

From Oroville on CA 70, take Exit 46, Oroville Dam Boulevard. Drive east 1.7 miles and turn right onto Olive Highway (CA 162). Drive east 6.3 miles and turn right onto Forbestown Road (signed to Forbestown). After 14 miles, continue straight onto Challenge Cut-Off Road, then go almost 3 miles to a junction with La Porte Road. Turn left, toward La Porte. Drive east on La Porte Road (Forest Service Road 120) 24 miles to La Porte. Continue east 2 miles, into Little Grass Valley Reservoir area, to a junction where La Porte Road breaks to the right, but instead continue straight 1 more mile, now on Little Grass Valley Road. Turn right at the sign marked PENINSULA RECREATION FACILITIES and proceed 0.5 mile. Bear right past the parking area for the boat launch, following the small sign to Wyandotte. Continue another 0.3 mile, then turn left into the campground.

GPS COORDINATES: N39° 43.642' W120° 59.063'

43

⛺ Upper Jamison Campground

Beauty ★★★★ / Privacy ★★★★ / Spaciousness ★★★★ / Quiet ★★★ / Security ★★★★★ / Cleanliness ★★★★

An experience in style and gentility—only the bears are rowdy.

Drive into Mohawk Valley on your way to Upper Jamison Campground, and all of a sudden you are in the land of lush green golf courses and condos. Graeagle, just 5 miles from the park, is a retirement mecca, with elegant restaurants, a good grocery store, a deli with smoked meats, and a pond with a great swimming beach right in the center of town.

The nearby Feather River Inn used to be the most fashionable resort in Northern California. Passengers arrived on the train, and porters pushed their steamer trunks over in wheelbarrows. Now the flannels and black cocktail dresses with pearls have given way to ski parkas or golf shirts, depending on the season, but the area still has a sense of style and gentility.

Drive into Plumas-Eureka State Park. The rangers are polite and friendly. Everything is tasteful and under control. The museum is thoughtfully done. The handout pamphlets are grammatically correct. Drive another mile or so to the Upper Jamison Campground at the end of the road. By pretty Little Jamison Creek, the campsites are well separated and nicely screened from one another by trees. The bathrooms are rough but clean. The whole camping experience is enjoyable, though a little removed. Maybe it's the area's rich history that gives you the Westminster Abbey feeling of strolling among the bones of kings and commoners whose hopes, dreams, and sins are now all dust.

Little Jamison Creek provides a nice ambience as it runs through Upper Jamison Campground.

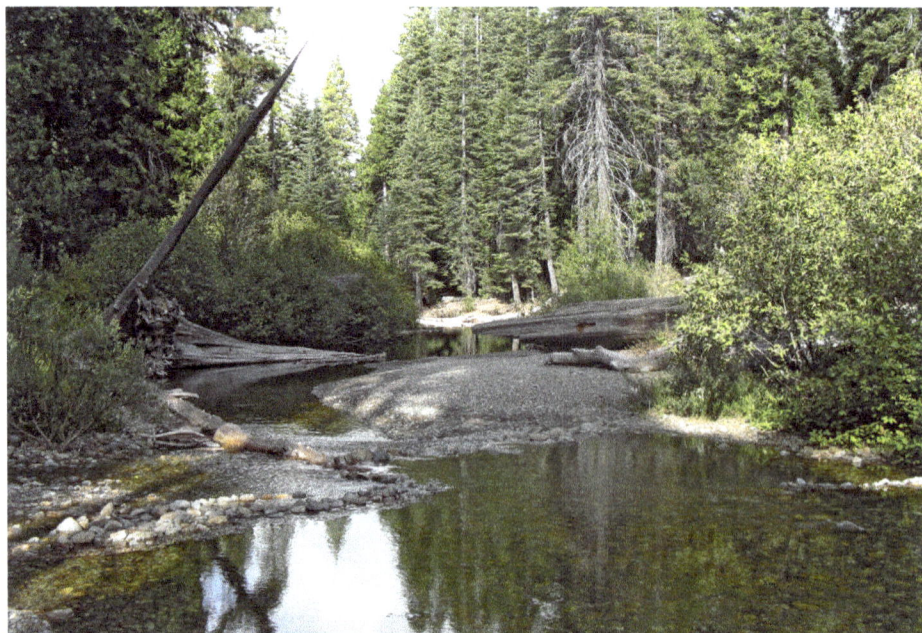

photographed by John Conway

KEY INFORMATION

LOCATION: 310 Johnsville Road, Blairsden, CA 96103

OPERATED BY: Plumas-Eureka State Park

CONTACT: 530-836-2380; www.parks. ca.gov

OPEN: May–late September

SITES: 67 sites for tents, trailers, or RVs, 14 walk-in sites

EACH SITE HAS: Picnic table, fireplace, food locker

ASSIGNMENT: First come, first-served; reservations recommended Memorial Day–Labor Day

REGISTRATION: At office in museum by entrance; reserve at 800-444-7275 or reservecalifornia.com

AMENITIES: Water, flush toilets, hot showers, wood for sale, wheelchair-accessible camping

PARKING: At individual site

FEE: $35, $8 extra vehicle

ELEVATION: 5,200'

RESTRICTIONS:

PETS: On leash only

FIRES: In fireplace

ALCOHOL: No restrictions

VEHICLES: RVs up to 28 feet, trailers up to 24 feet

OTHER: No burning of dead or downed wood—purchased firewood only

Indeed, except for nearby Jamison City's (now Johnsville) brief raffish period replete with fisticuffs and fancy women, the area has always been respectable. Johnsville was a mining town with solid citizens brought in from Wales, Austria, and elsewhere to work the mines and live in harmony (and now all buried in the local Johnsville cemetery—worth a visit).

Only the bears are rude. Folks are implored to cooperate with the rangers to keep those naughty ursines in line. Don't leave food around while you are not in the area. Keep a clean camp. Put your food and coolers in your trunk when you do leave. If you have a hatchback, disguise the coolers with a blanket or haphazardly placed clothes. Bears are smart, strong, and very hungry. They have been known to tear open an automobile like a sardine can just to get a tube of sunscreen.

Naturally, we were there for two days and didn't see a bear. We did see the work of beavers up at Madora Lake, as well as Canada geese, coots, and a glimpse of what might have been a fox around dusk on our walk. Directions to Madora Lake are quite clear in the Plumas-Eureka State Park handout. In fact, you passed the turnoff to the lake on your way in from Graeagle.

Walking in and around Madora Lake takes about an hour. On the far side of the lake is a picnic table, perfect for a sandwich or a sundowner while you look for beaver. This industrious rodent practically fueled the Western exploration. During the late 1700s and early 1800s, explorers headed west as they decimated the Eastern beaver population. They cured the pelts and sent them to factories where the hair was made into felt, which was then made into beaver top hats. These hats held their shape, repelled water, and were all the rage for a while.

Now the beavers have aggressively bounced back and can be seen around Plumas-Eureka State Park (another beaver-sighting hot spot is Lake Earl Wildlife Area just north of Crescent City). Beavers like streams around aspen, birch, alder, and willow. They come out most in the summer after the birth of their kits and work mainly in the early morning and evening.

Another great hike is up the Grass Lake Trail, where you will find even more beaver signs. Grass Lake is pretty and surrounded by Jeffrey pine and red fir. Work your way around to the west side of the lake to get the best view of the incredible mountains on the other side.

Don't miss camping at Plumas-Eureka; it's a real treasure. And on your way out or in, don't miss The Brewing Lair, a small, mostly outdoor microbrewery in Blairsden along CA 70. Folks of all ages enjoy Ping-Pong, Cornhole, slacklining, and just relaxing on the rolling, shaded hillside with a freshly brewed pint.

Upper Jamison Campground

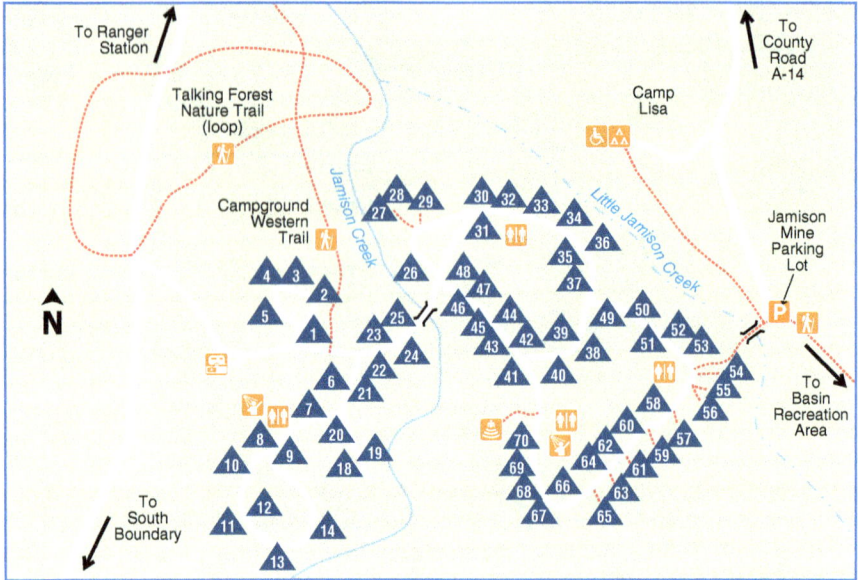

GETTING THERE

From Graeagle, take CA 89 north to CA 70. Take CA 70 west to County Road A14 and go 5 miles to Plumas-Eureka State Park. Go left past the park headquarters to the campground at the end of the road.

GPS COORDINATES: N39° 44.427' W120° 42.430'

44

Haskins Valley Campground

Beauty ★★★★★ / Privacy ★★★ / Spaciousness ★★★ / Quiet ★★★ / Security ★★★ / Cleanliness ★★★★

This is easy summer camping, with lazy afternoons of reading novels and fishing on the lake.

Here's another beautiful campground in Pacific Gas & Electric (PG&E) land. As usual, the campground is well conceived and well tended. PG&E is mindful of its image and sets out to curry favor with the public, to make up for those times when it has to draw down the level of its reservoirs in late summer to satisfy us energy guzzlers in the flatland below. That's when folks look around and say, "Hey, Bucks Lake isn't a lake at all but a reservoir contained by a dam. And Haskins Valley is named for the valley where the lake is now."

Still, I love Bucks Lake, Haskins Valley Campground, and electric lights, in that order. The sites are set on a handsome pined knoll embraced by the lake. All you see is the waving green of the pines and the sparkling blue-green sky and water. What a spot to spend a week! This is kick-back-and-relax country. Quincy is just down the road, so you don't have to worry about serious supplies. There is a store right on the lake that sells sundries. In Meadow Valley below, the road splits to make a low road and a high road to Bucks Lake. Take the 2-mile-longer low option, Big Creek Road, if you don't trust your ancient automobile (and admire incredible dogwoods). At Bucks Lake, you'll find boats to rent,

Campers at Haskins Valley can get out on the water with a boat rental from Bucks Lake Marina. The marina has pontoon, fishing, and ski boat rentals as well as kayaks and canoes.

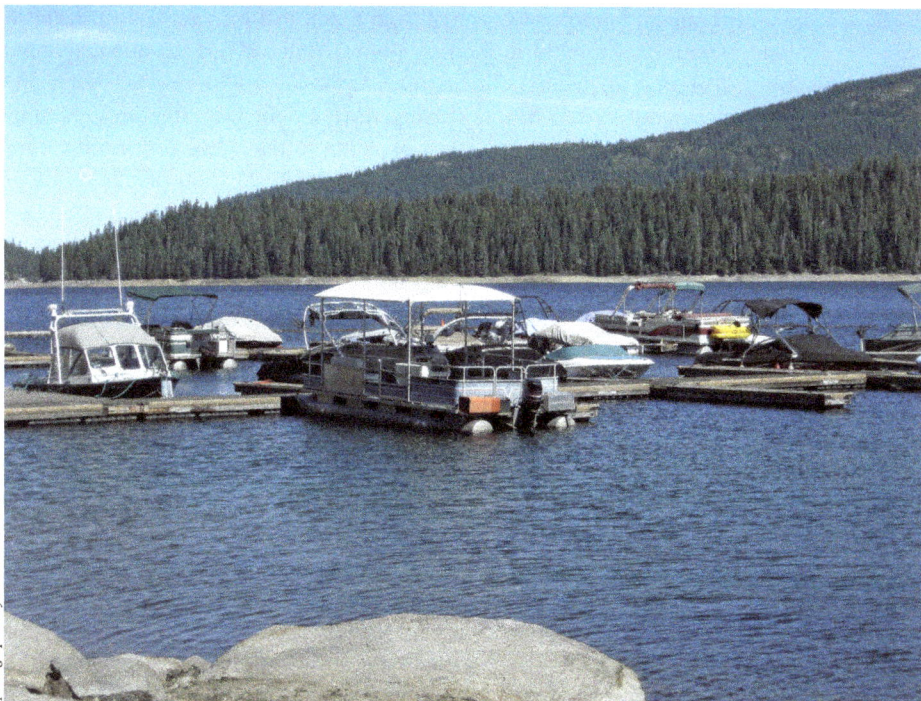

photographed by Kummerle/Flickr

KEY INFORMATION

LOCATION: 16731 Bucks Lake Road, Quincy, CA 95971

OPERATED BY: Pacific Gas & Electric

CONTACT: 916-386-5164; recreation.pge.com

OPEN: Mid-May–mid-October (weather permitting)

SITES: 65 total: 5 tent sites; 60 sites for tents, RVs, and trailers

EACH SITE HAS: Picnic table, fireplace, barbecue

ASSIGNMENT: First come, first served; reservations available for most sites

REGISTRATION: At entrance

AMENITIES: Water, vault toilets

PARKING: At individual site

FEE: $25, $5 extra vehicle

ELEVATION: 5,200'

RESTRICTIONS:

PETS: On leash only

FIRES: In fireplace

ALCOHOL: No restrictions

VEHICLES: RVs and trailers allowed (no hookups)

OTHER: Don't leave food out

shoreline to explore, hikes to take, and a lake that warms up in summer to temperatures that suit even the most spoiled swimmer.

Think summer camping: bring a tent you can stand up in—and sit in your folding chair. Consider a screen house too, as there are voracious mosquitoes in this area; out there when the bloodsuckers are buzzing in your ears, a screen house is worth its weight in gold. The last time I was out at Bucks Lake, I complained about the mosquitoes and heard the polite laughter of an elderly couple a campsite away who were sitting genteelly inside their screen house around a card table. I found that Coleman sold a minimal version, and I bought it. Now I'm looking forward to sitting in it, reading a novel, and listening to unenlightened campers slapping skeeters.

Bucks Lake is heavy-duty cross-country-skiing territory. In fact, this area, notably Johnsville, takes credit for introducing the sport of skiing to the West. Apparently, miners from Norway and Sweden built "long boards" or "snowshoes" from planks up to 12 feet long, weighing about 20 pounds. Now we call them skis. The miners used them to get around in deep snow—for fun, they started downhill races above Eureka Lake. According to legend, they reached up to 80 miles per hour; a long ski pole held between the legs was used as a brake or as a pivot.

Quincy is a fun visit. Looking like a movie set for the all-American town, it is the Plumas County seat and home to the Plumas County Museum, which chronicles Quincy's involvement with gold mining, logging, and the railroad. Imagine the wives arriving from the East to join their gold-miner husbands at Quincy. One wrote, "Our fare is very plain, consisting of meat and bread, bread and meat, now and then some rancid butter that was put up in the Land Of Goshen [the East] and sent on a six-month cruise by Cape Horn, for which we give the sum of $2 a pound." Of course, all this on top of crude log cabins, rowdy forty-niners, and the heartbreak of betting your all on striking it rich.

The museum also has a decent exhibit on the Maidu Indians, the previous leaseholders of the area that includes Plumas County (named for bird feathers a Spanish explorer observed in the river). The Maidu, who ironically never valued gold, did use gold-laced quartz for spear tips, knives, and mortars. They were low-key American Indians who "trod very lightly" on the land and at first gazed with curiosity at the forty-niners and their industrious ways. For a while, the Maidu were happy to find gold to trade with the white man for a shirt or a pair of pantaloons. Soon enough, however, the two groups collided, and the Maidu passed rapidly into history.

When you drive around Quincy, look at the trees—the impressive oak, maple, and poplar. Quincy folks were loggers, and they knew their trees. Look for the Morning Thunder Cafe—good breakfast. Then drive up Bucks Lake Road—11 miles to the Bucks Summit Trailhead—and climb your calories off ascending the southern flank of Mount Pleasant.

Haskins Valley Campground

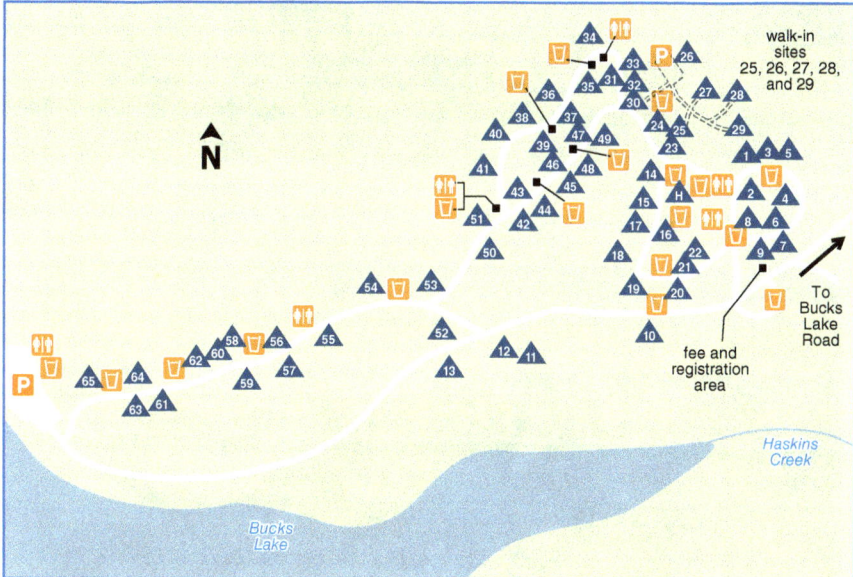

GETTING THERE

From Quincy, turn west on Bucks Lake Road, and drive 16.5 miles to the campground.

GPS COORDINATES: N39° 52.200' W121° 10.445'

YOSEMITE

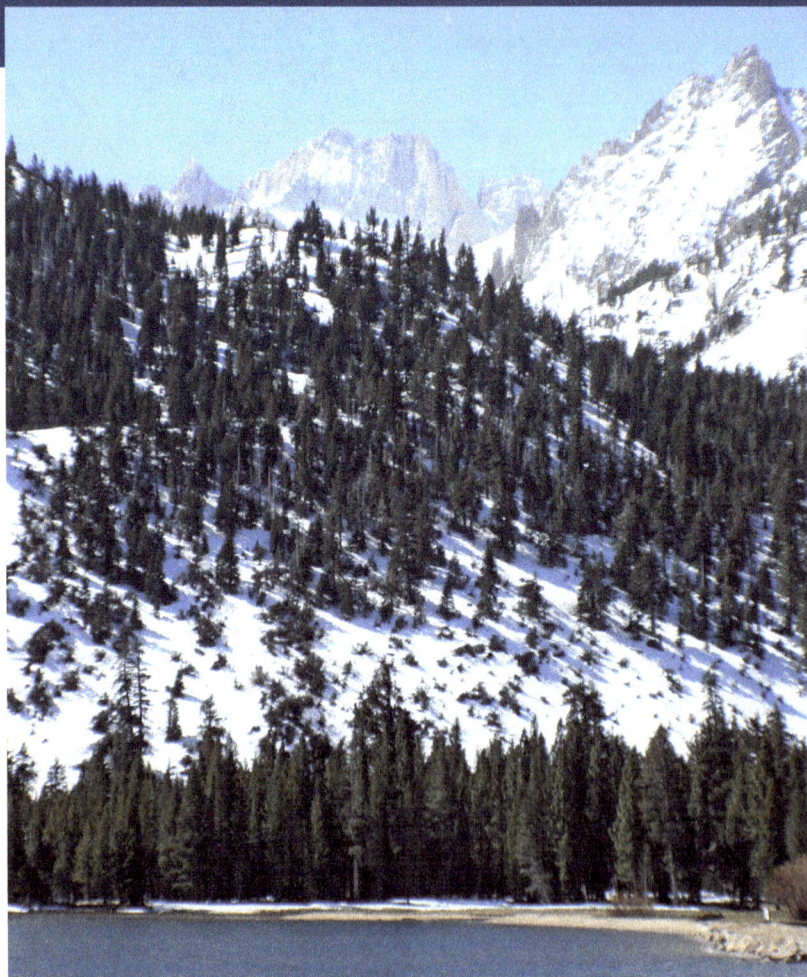

Matterhorn (12,280') and Sawtooth Ridge (11,980') Peaks are a striking backdrop to Twin Lakes, a short jaunt from Buckeye Campground *(see page 172)*.

45

Twin Lakes Campground

Beauty ★★★★★ / Privacy ★★★★ / Spaciousness ★★★★★ / Quiet ★★★ / Security ★★★★★ / Cleanliness ★★★★★

The perfect place to spend summer vacation with the family.

The Twin Lakes around this campground look like blue beans joined at the hip. A little bridge connects the two lakes, and folks in rental rowboats and canoes scoot underneath it. Grandfathers teach their grandchildren how to fish as a waterfall cascades down the cliff above the lakes.

The campground is both accessible and friendly. There are rustic cabins, a lodge, and a store. A few miles away, in the city of Mammoth Lakes, you'll find pizzerias, hardware stores, and a big, wonderful Vons Supermarket on Old Mammoth Road. Twin Lakes Campground is a great place to camp for a week; bring your family for the summer vacation.

The campsites sprawl around the two lakes and uphill across the road. If Twin Lakes Campground doesn't have any reservations available, consider beautiful Coldwater Campground on Coldwater Creek just a few miles up the road. Or try Lake Mary and Lake George Campgrounds just a mile or so up the road. All the sites are wonderful but often not as popular as the ones at Twin Lakes. Phone the rangers to check on site availability, and plan your trip so you arrive either in off-season or by Thursday for the weekend.

Rent and launch fishing boats on idyllic Twin Lakes right from the general store.

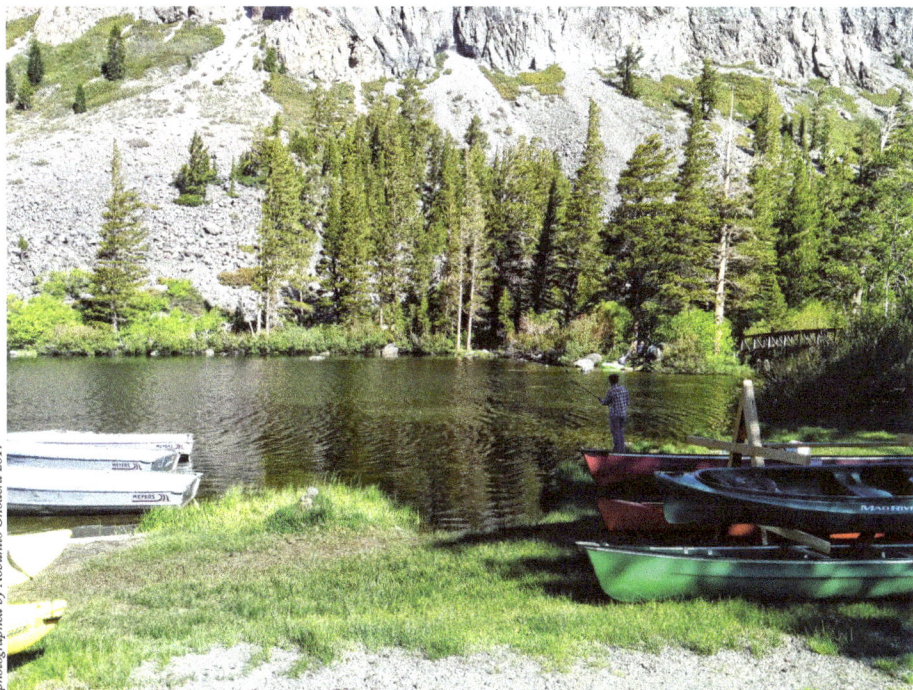

photographed by Nobuhito Onodera 2017

KEY INFORMATION

LOCATION: 518 Twin Lakes Road, Mammoth Lakes, CA 93546

OPERATED BY: Inyo National Forest, Mammoth Ranger District

CONTACT: 760-924-5500; www.fs.usda.gov /inyo

OPEN: May 25–late October

SITES: 94

EACH SITE HAS: Picnic table, fireplace, food locker

ASSIGNMENT: First come, first served; reservations available

REGISTRATION: At entrance; reserve at 877-444-6777 or recreation.gov

AMENITIES: Water, flush toilets, boat rental, 4 wheelchair-accessible sites

PARKING: At individual site

FEE: $23, $7 extra vehicle

ELEVATION: 8,600'

RESTRICTIONS:

PETS: On leash only

FIRES: In fireplaces

ALCOHOL: No restrictions

VEHICLES: RVs up to 48 feet

OTHER: Store all food and scented items in food lockers. To reduce vehicle traffic into the Devils Postpile area, a shuttle system has been implemented. Hikers pay a fee to use the shuttle; campers can enter with a car but need to pay an entry fee (in addition to the camping fee). Leaving your car at your campsite and using the shuttle is highly encouraged. Stop at the Mammoth Lakes visitor center (on the right side of CA 203 on the way into Mammoth Lakes) or the Adventure Center (at the ski area) for more information.

Head to the top of Coldwater Campground and walk a few hundred yards to the old Mammoth Consolidated Gold Mine on Mineral Hill. Here you can see some of the old buildings from the mining towns and locations of the many bawdy houses and a saloon named The Temple of Folly (long since destroyed). Walk around the old buildings and rusted machinery and imagine the men who sweated in the summer sun and froze in the winter, obsessed with gold. Climb up to the upper adit in the early morning for a view of Mount Banner and Mount Ritter.

Take the nice little hike to Emerald Lake. It's about a mile up the mountain. The trailhead and parking lot are next to the parking lot for the mine on Mineral Hill. Walk up by Coldwater Creek, where there are lupine, monkey flower, and fireweed. Bring a picnic and climb the rocks around the lake. Bring fishing gear as well. I watched one woman reel in two decent trout while I ate my sandwich.

If you are ambitious, go around the left side of Emerald Lake. At the signed junction, go right to Gentian Meadow–Sky Meadows. Climb up by the inlet creek and reach tiny Gentian Meadow. Carry on up past a waterfall, and after a while you'll reach Sky Meadows. Look for paintbrush, corn lily, and elephant's-head among the grass. It's about 2.5 miles back down the hill.

Or if you are truly ambitious, pick up the trail to Duck Pass (8.2 miles round-trip) back in the parking lot by the trailhead to Emerald Lake. Find the Duck Pass sign, and start climbing. When you reach the entry sign for the John Muir Wilderness, bear right. Climb up through lodgepoles, pines, and hemlocks, and carry on past the trail to Arrowhead Lake, Skelton Lake, and Barney Lake. Next you'll see alpine Duck Pass ahead, with all the high-elevation flowers—columbine, gentian, and sorrel. Finally, traverse the pass and you'll see Duck Lake and pretty little Pika Lake on the left.

Back at Twin Lakes Campground, a nice stroll is around the shore to the falls. Access the trail behind campsite 37. You'll see a sign that says PRIVATE ROAD. Bear left and follow the trail that heads through the trees to the waterfall. Or walk over to Tamarack Lodge. This graceful establishment was built in 1923. The clerk from the grocery store averred that Tamarack Lodge has the best food in Mammoth Lakes.

However, we ate chez campsite the last time I was at Twin Lakes. I boiled some quartered potatoes and set them aside. Then I fried some onions, garlic, jalapeño peppers, and strips of chicken breast in the pot. After a bit, I returned the potatoes to the pot and stirred it all about. Very delicious for a one-pot meal!

About 3:15 a.m., I heard a visitor. I jumped out of my sleeping bag and poked my head out of the tent. A 3-foot bear was rifling through my cooler of soft drinks. I shouted, and the midget bear looked at me insolently and pawed on. I threw a pebble, and he ran over to a tree and climbed up a few feet. I retrieved my cooler. He gave me the evil eye and ran into the underbrush. The next morning he was rooting around in the big trash container down by the bridge. He glared at me and sauntered off, combing garbage out of his whiskers.

Twin Lakes Campground

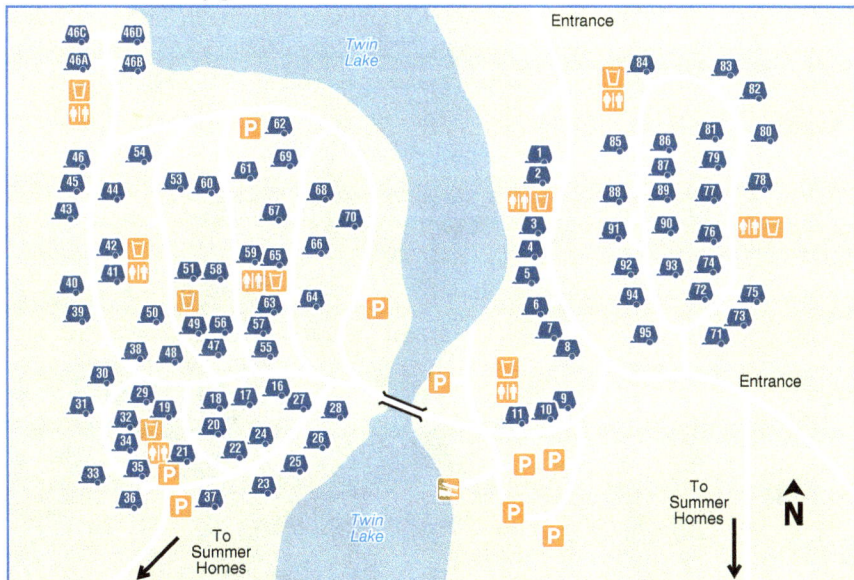

GETTING THERE

Take US 395 to Mammoth Lakes. From US 395, head west on CA 203, which will become Main Street and then Lake Mary Road, for a total of 6 miles. Veer right and follow Twin Lakes Road about a mile to the campground.

GPS COORDINATES: N37° 36.950' W119° 0.416'

46

⚠ Minaret Falls Campground

Beauty ★★★★★ / Privacy ★★★ / Spaciousness ★★★★★ / Quiet ★★★★★ / Security ★★★★★ / Cleanliness ★★★★

The prettiest in a string of beautiful, popular campgrounds on the Upper San Joaquin River

When you drive down the dirt road into the campground, silvery Minaret Falls leaps out at you. On my last visit, even in late September the water cascaded down the mountainside like streams of crystal.

Right away, we drove into a campsite with a clean and soft tent pitch shrouded by trees. Through the willows we could see the riverbank and the falls.

We drove a few miles up the road to Red's Meadow store and café to buy worms and salmon eggs for trout fishing. A little bear was raiding the back room of the store, but the clerk and a tourist scared him away. A dog lunged at the end of his leash, barking at the curious animal as he scurried off. We learned that the original Red was a gold miner who turned to tourism when the Depression and falling gold prices drove him out of business. His pack station at Red's Meadow was one of the first tourist draws in the Mammoth area.

We hiked the 1.25 miles down to Rainbow Falls, along with a passel of other folks. We took the rough stairs down to the exquisite falls and stood in the spray. A rainbow arced through the mist.

The 366-mile San Joaquin River originates in the Ansel Adams Wilderness and flows alongside Minaret Falls Campground on its way to the Central Valley.

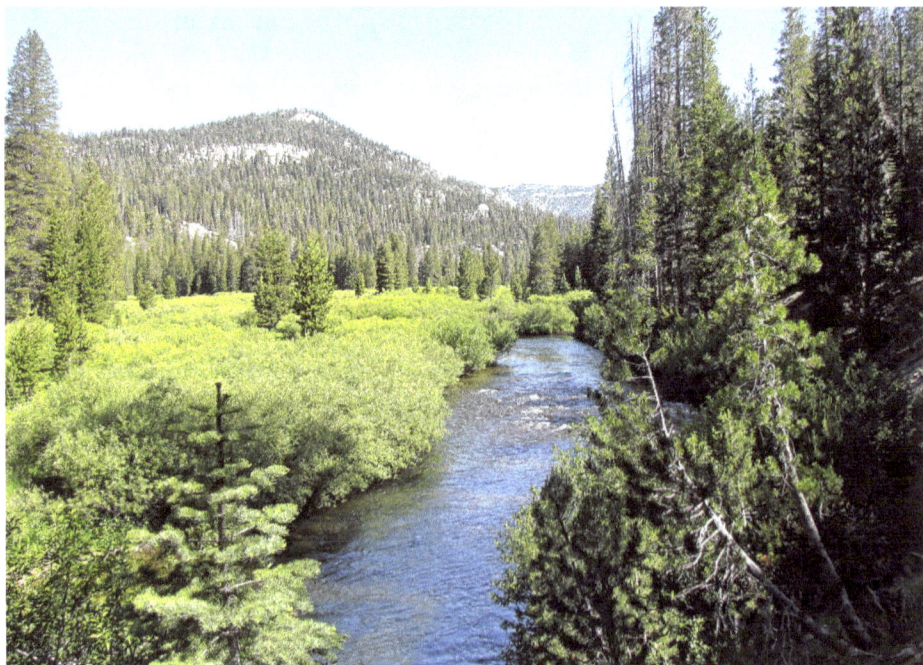

photographed by Lori Long

KEY INFORMATION

LOCATION: Minaret Summit Road, 1.5 miles from Devils Postpile National Monument, Mammoth Lakes, CA 93546

OPERATED BY: Inyo National Forest, Mammoth Ranger District

CONTACT: 760-924-5500, www.fs.usda.gov /inyo

OPEN: Mid-June–September

SITES: 27

EACH SITE HAS: Picnic table, fireplace, food locker

ASSIGNMENT: First come, first served; no reservations

REGISTRATION: At entrance

AMENITIES: Water, vault toilets

PARKING: At individual site

FEE: $23, $7 extra vehicle

ELEVATION: 7,600'

RESTRICTIONS:

PETS: On leash only

FIRES: In fireplace

ALCOHOL: No restrictions

VEHICLES: RVs up to 22 feet

OTHER: No dispersed camping in this area; 14-day stay limit; store food and scented items in food lockers. Note: To reduce vehicle traffic in the Devils Postpile area, a shuttle system has been implemented. Hikers pay a fee to use the shuttle; campers can enter with a car but must pay an entry fee (in addition to the camping fee). Leaving your car at your campsite and using the shuttle is highly encouraged. Stop at the Mammoth Lakes visitor center (on the right side of CA 203 on the way into Mammoth Lakes) or the Adventure Center (at the ski area) for more information.

We hiked back through an area of firs, lodgepoles, and Jeffrey pines, scarred, like most of Devils Postpile National Monument, by a 1992 wildfire. Following the fire, rangers walked through the burn to assess the damage, and charred trees crashed down around them. It wasn't safe to walk there for months.

Back at Minaret Campground we floated salmon eggs and earthworms down the river and caught six trout. We wrapped them in aluminum foil with herbs and cooked them over the campfire. It was a gorgeous night. The southern Sierras have hundreds of shooting stars.

Sleeping that night in our tent, I heard the rustle of a visitor—a bear. He ran away when I got up, and I inspected the damage. My two treasured inflatable sinks, which we use to wash the dishes, were ruined. The bear had bitten a big hole in each of them. To add insult to injury, he also bit into my plastic collapsible water jug. Were these acts of rancor, or did he think they were full of food?

A neighbor came over. The bear had tried to open the hatch of his Nissan Z; the telltale paw marks gave the intruder away. I told him about my sinks. He recommended wiping sinks, picnic tables, and cooler tops each night with bleach. Bears like soap, but they don't like bleach. I went back to my sleeping bag and heard the bear slouch through the camp again.

The next morning we walked north along the river and crossed on a log at the end of the campground. There's a short trail to the foot of Minaret Falls. We bushwhacked up to the top of the falls and dipped in some nice pools.

Later, we hiked up to Shadow Lake. It's no easy climb (round-trip is about 7 miles), but you'll agree it's worth it when you see beautiful blue Shadow Lake against huge, craggy Mount Ritter. To find the trailhead, take the shuttle toward Mammoth from Minaret Falls Campground to the road to Agnew Meadows Campground. About 0.3 mile in, you'll find trailhead parking with toilets and drinking water. Take the River Trail and follow the signs to Shadow Lake, through another parking lot and across a creek to another trail junction at about 1 mile. To the left is Reds Meadow. To the right is Shadow Lake. With Mammoth Mountain at your back, climb past Olaine Lake, cross the San Joaquin River on a wooden bridge, and hump it up the canyon wall to Shadow Lake. You'll find good fishing, so bring your fishing gear and bait.

Minaret Falls Campground is popular. Be sure to phone rangers ahead of time to make sure it's open and see how crowded it will be. Try to plan a trip before or after the prime summertime season and arrive on Thursday if you want to spend the weekend. The area is so popular that during the summer, hikers (not campers) are required to park their cars at the Mammoth Ski Resort and take the intravalley shuttle down.

You have 30 minutes from the time you occupy a campsite to pay. Park your car at the first empty campsite you find, and use that 30 minutes to walk around and see if you like another site better. If you find one, leave something on the picnic table, and go move your car.

Minaret Falls Campground

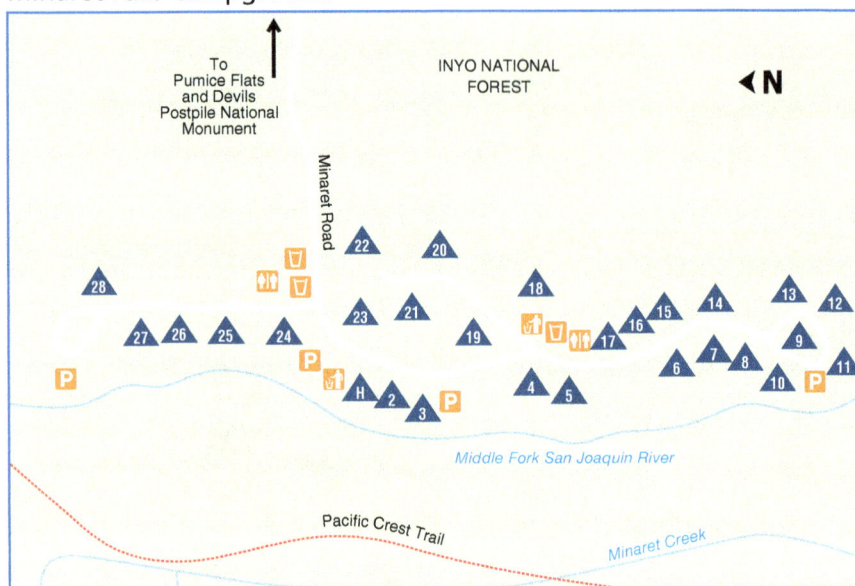

GETTING THERE

Take US 395 to Mammoth Lakes. From US 395, drive 4 miles west on Main Street/CA 203. Turn right onto Minaret Road/CA 203 and continue 13 miles to the campground.

GPS COORDINATES: N37° 38.417' W119° 5.005'

47

Benton Hot Springs Campground

Beauty ★★★★ / Privacy ★★★ / Spaciousness ★★★★ / Quiet ★★★★ / Security ★★★★★ /
Cleanliness ★★★★

Unparalleled stargazing from your very own private hot tub in the heart of the Wild West

Mammoth Lakes and the surrounding areas overflow with outdoor recreation opportunities. Tall, voluminous mountains draped in wintry white blankets become lush oases for summer camping. Sapphire lakes sparkle, lively creeks tumble over granite boulders, and hordes of people coming from every direction jockey for a piece of wilderness to call home for a night.

But then you hear about Benton Hot Springs, just shy of 40 miles east of Mammoth and US 395, and it sounds intriguing. East, you say, an incredulous tone in your voice. What could possibly be east of Mammoth? Nevada?

Yes, there is Nevada, but before the state line is Benton Hot Springs—an oasis, a time capsule, and a worthy camping destination for folks who like their adventures seriously off the beaten path. There is nobody out here, just you, whomever you dragged along with you, and about a billion stars. This is the ancient home of the Ute Ute Gwaitu Paiute Tribe, or the "Hot Water Place People." The Ute Ute were drawn into the Blind Springs Valley by the natural springs that bubble to the earth's surface at 140°F and carve a steamy stream on the southern border of what is now the campground.

It's all about the view at Benton Hot Springs Campground, where the alpenglow turns the White Mountains gold at sunset and the skies come alive with stars at night.

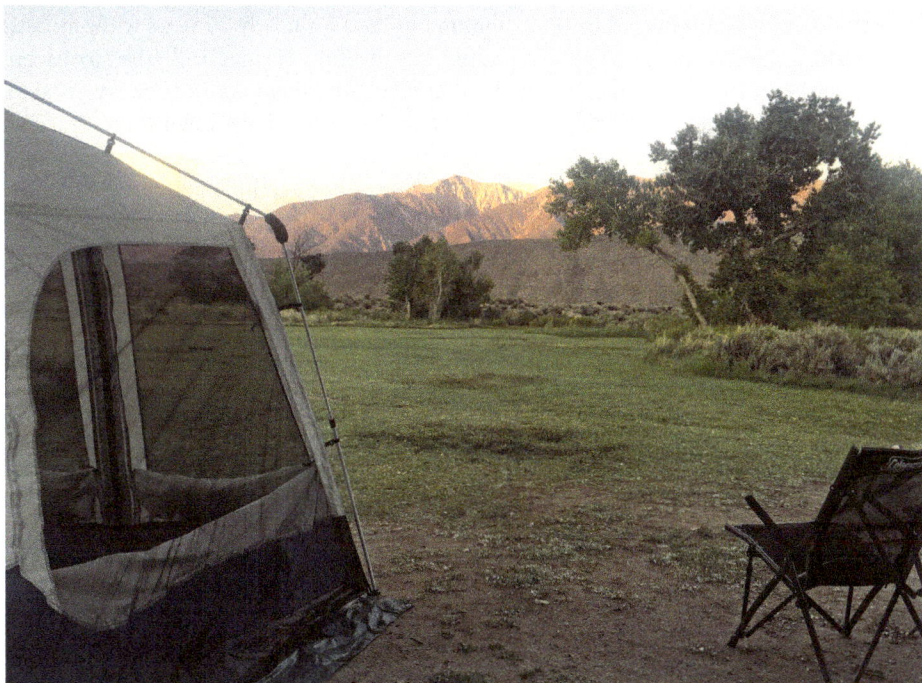

KEY INFORMATION

LOCATION: 55137 CA 120, Benton, CA 93512

OPERATED BY: Bramlette Family Trust

CONTACT: 760-933-2287, 866-466-2824; bentonhotsprings.org

OPEN: Year-round

SITES: 11 sites for tents or RVs

EACH SITE HAS: Picnic table, fire pit, private hot tub

ASSIGNMENT: By phone or submit request online; from bentonhotsprings.org, click on "Hot Tubs" then "Reservations"

REGISTRATION: At the Inn at Benton Hot Springs

AMENITIES: Water, vault toilets

PARKING: At individual site

FEE: Sites 1–3: $50, double occupancy; sites 4–11: $60, triple occupancy; $10 additional person

ELEVATION: 5,630'

RESTRICTIONS:

PETS: Well-behaved pets allowed

FIRES: In fire pit

ALCOHOL: No restrictions

VEHICLES: No length limit

OTHER: No music allowed

This is not your usual state-park camping. First off, the grounds are privately owned and operated, in conjunction with a kitschy bed-and-breakfast, by the Bramlette family and have been since Buster and MaBelle built what was then the Wai Wera Motel in the mid-1900s. Before that, Dora A. Clausen ran the successful Conway boardinghouse in the mid-1800s. The house, circa 1865, still stands and hosts visitors. In fact, many of Benton's silver mining–era structures still stand. Fork over $5 for the informative pamphlet "A Walk Around Old Benton," and take a self-guided walking tour of the town's two dozen historical sites.

After silver was discovered in 1862, Benton boomed for nearly 25 years while an estimated $10 million in precious metals poured out of Blind Springs Hill. The stories are fascinating: in a town that once boasted 5,000 residents, there was a brewery; a jail; a Chinatown; and enough gunfights, house fires, and murders for a town three times its size. Today, it's not quite a ghost town.

Lose yourself in the Wild West or the high desert; both compete for your attention. Sweeping views to the east of the magnificent White Mountain range and its multiple peaks exceeding 13,000 feet grace every one of the small campground's 11 sites, making for unforgettable sunrises and sunsets. A closer look into this barren, rocky range reveals herds of bighorn sheep and even wild mustangs. If that's your thing, you can book a four-night guided ride into the wilderness north of Boundary Peak and see these majestic animals from the seat of your saddle (888-9-TRAILS [872-457]; hiddentrails.com).

In the campground, jackrabbits scamper between the sage tufts. Western tanagers and red-winged blackbirds perch in the bushes. And the dry air, combined with some of the least light-polluted skies in the country, yields unparalleled stargazing from your very own hot tub.

Yes, that's right: probably the most unique aspect of Benton is that each of the sites boasts a private hot tub piped with water from the natural hot-springs creek flowing alongside the campground. Two sites, shaded by towering cottonwood groves, even offer creekside camping. All of the sites are massive and offer a certain degree of privacy, but aside from the small cottonwood grove, there isn't too much in the way of shade. Bring your sunblock and make sure to stake down the tent, as winds are known to barrel through this campground any time of year. Bug spray is also a must, as the thirsty resident mosquitoes have somehow adapted to the heavy winds and bite in all kinds of conditions.

For a heart-pumping hike (2,000 feet up in 1.4 miles) head to Glass Mountain, Mono County's highest point at 11,129 feet, offering breathtaking views in all directions. Glass Mountain lies on the northeast corner of the Long Valley Caldera, the largest of its kind in North America. Around 760,000 years ago, a massive eruption of the Long Valley volcano formed the caldera and sent debris flying into the sky as far as Nebraska.

From Benton, drive 13.6 miles west on CA 120, and turn south onto Black Canyon Road. After 0.8 mile bear west (right) on Sawmill Meadows Road, and in another 6.6 miles turn left to stay on Sawmill Meadows Road. Keep right in 3.2 miles to stay on a jeep road, which eventually leads to the trailhead.

Benton Hot Springs Campground

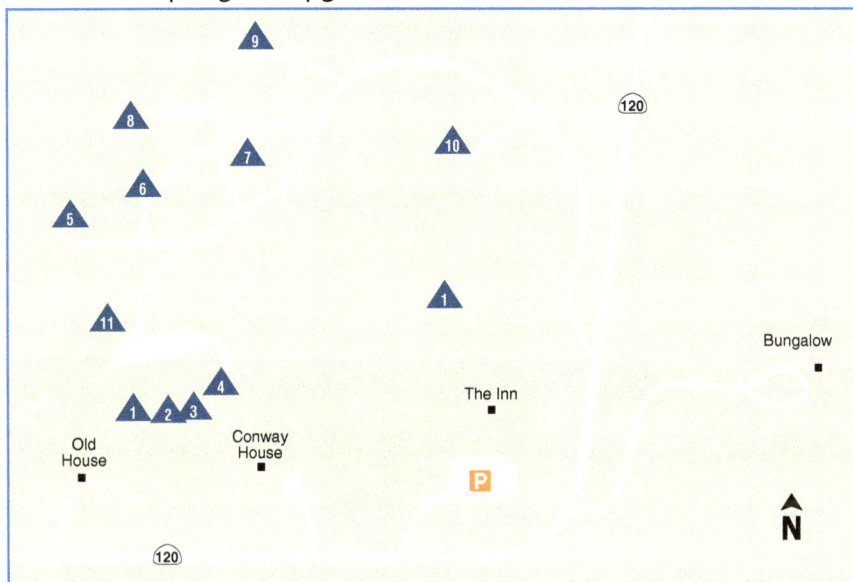

GETTING THERE

From the intersection of US 395 and CA 120 in Lee Vining, head south 5.3 miles, and turn left onto CA 120. Go 41.6 miles, and the campground will be on your left.

GPS COORDINATES: N37° 48.052' W118° 31.687'

48

White Wolf Campground

Beauty ★★★★★ / Privacy ★★★★★ / Spaciousness ★★★★★ / Quiet ★★★★★ / Security ★★★★★ / Cleanliness ★★★★★

The only campground in Yosemite National Park worth squeezing into

Yosemite National Park is heaven on earth. With the Mariposa Battalion, the first English-speaking party to see Yosemite Valley, was Lafayette Bunnell. He wrote: "The grandeur of the scene was softened by the haze that hung over the valley—light as gossamer—and by the clouds which partially dimmed the higher cliffs and mountains. This obscurity of vision merely increased the awe with which I beheld it, and as I looked, a peculiar exalted sensation seemed to fill my whole being, and I found my eyes in tears with emotion."

The Yosemite Indians, the original inhabitants, loved the valley too, but the arrival of the forty-niners ended their resiliency. By 1852 Chief Tenaya of the Yosemites, his tribe decimated, was stoned to death by some raiding Mono Indians. Soon after, August T. Dowd, a miner hunting in the valley, saw a tree bigger than he'd ever seen before. He told his friends about it, and the tourists began flooding in. Yosemite Valley became a mecca to the world.

Now, 4-hour traffic jams in Yosemite Valley are common, and the campgrounds are constantly booked. Avoid Yosemite Valley and explore the rest of the park instead. Come in

Wildflowers flourish in the wet meadows and riverbanks surrounding White Wolf Campground. Don't forget the bug spray!

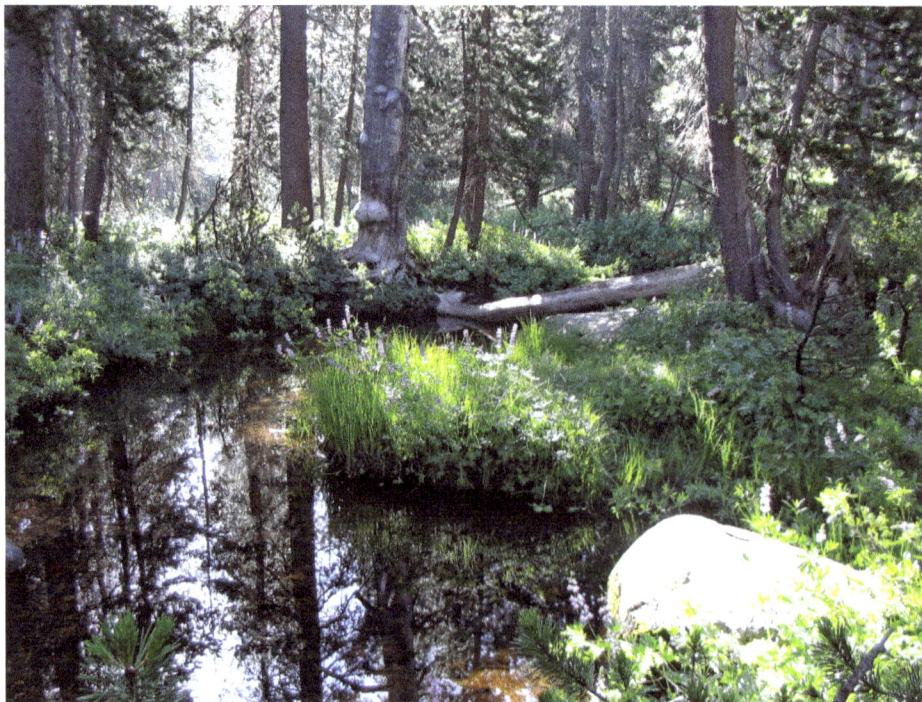

photographed by Jeff Goddard

KEY INFORMATION

LOCATION: Off Tioga Road (CA 120) about 1 hour north of Yosemite Valley, Yosemite National Park, CA 95389

OPERATED BY: Yosemite National Park

CONTACT: 209-372-0200; nps.gov/yose

OPEN: July–late September (depending on road and weather conditions); if gate is locked, the grounds are closed; opens after last snow

SITES: 74 sites for RVs and tents

EACH SITE HAS: Fire ring, picnic table, food locker

ASSIGNMENT: First come, first served; no reservations

REGISTRATION: At entrance

AMENITIES: Water, flush toilets

PARKING: At individual site

FEE: $18

ELEVATION: 8,000'

RESTRICTIONS:

PETS: On leash only

FIRES: In fireplace

ALCOHOL: No restrictions

VEHICLES: RVs up to 27 feet; trailers up to 24 feet

OTHER: Don't leave food out; 14-day stay limit

from the east over the Tioga Pass off US 395 or from the west on CA 120. Shun CA 41, and don't get stuck in the Wawona Tunnel.

However, you should see Tuolumne Meadows and camp in White Wolf Campground. John Muir eloquently described the Tioga Pass area: "From garden to garden, ridge to ridge, I drifted enchanted, now on my knees gazing into the face of a daisy, now climbing again and again among the purple and azure flowers of the hemlocks, now down into the treasuries of the snow, or gazing far over domes and peaks, lakes and woods, and the billowy glaciated fields of the upper Tuolumne. In the midst of such beauty, pierced with its rays, one's body is all one tingling palate. Who wouldn't be a mountaineer! Up here all the world's prizes seem nothing."

White Wolf Campground is full of tiny meadows and stands of lodgepole pines, and the Middle Tuolumne River flows through the campground, which is constructed beautifully: The sites are set among the pines and granite boulders, and each loop seems miles away from the others. The arrangement of the tables and sites creates a sense of spaciousness. The facilities are clean and well tended. This is slow, elegant camping.

Only the little bear wandering around camp caused a little nervousness for us. Obviously it was a special bear because it had little colored tags in its ears. Our neighbor shook a towel at it, and it decamped, at least for that day. Of course, we were careful to put away our coolers even if we were only leaving camp for a moment. Bears get a record for raiding campers, and the rangers are forced to take steps. We didn't want that to happen to the little bear with tags in its ears.

We hiked up to Hardin Lake and sat under the pines, reading John Muir. Muir cavorted through these mountains, wearing a greatcoat and carrying all his gear in his pockets. At night, he lay down in the same massive coat and slept. Those old-timers were real men!

Take John A. "Snowshoe" Thompson, for example. Every winter from 1856 to 1876, Thompson carried the U.S. mail alone across the Sierra. Traveling on skis (called snowshoes in those days), Thompson carried a 100-pound pack and made the 180-mile round-trip in five days. His diet consisted of beef jerky and crackers, and he drank snow. He didn't carry a blanket or wear an overcoat.

At night, Thompson would find a tree stump. After setting fire to the stump, he'd cut some fir boughs for a bed. With his feet to the fire, he'd sleep through the worst blizzards. If he was caught outside camp in a bad blizzard, he would just stand on a rock and dance a jig to stay warm.

Today, camping life is a little easier. Still, remember to get supplies in the western flatlands or in Mammoth Lakes on your way in from the east. Ice, beer, soda, and a decent, fast food—style hot breakfast and lunch menu are available in Tuolumne Meadows, Crane Flat, and White Wolf Lodge near White Wolf Campground (in the summer months only).

White Wolf Campground

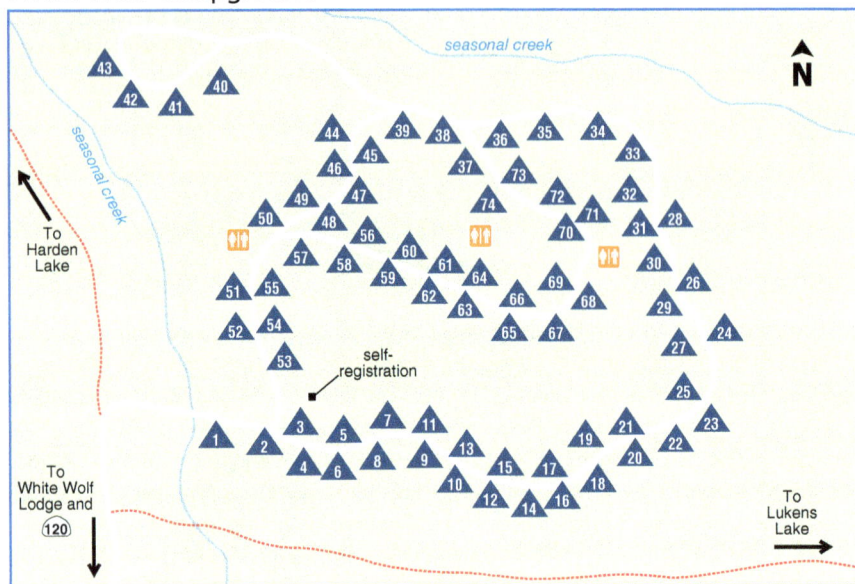

GETTING THERE

From US 395 in Lee Vining, take CA 120 (Tioga Road) west 43 miles to White Wolf Road on the right. The White Wolf Campground is about a mile down that road.

GPS COORDINATES: N37° 52.250' W119° 38.833'

49

⚘ Saddlebag Lake Campground

Beauty ★★★★ / Privacy ★★★ / Spaciousness ★★★★ / Quiet ★★★★★ / Security ★★★★★ /
Cleanliness ★★★★★

Perched on a knoll overlooking one of a series of jewel-like alpine lakes

The Sierra Nevada landscape is a pristine and dramatic mix of glacier-carved granite, snow-fed streams and lakes, wildflower-dotted meadows, and ancient forests; this is one of the most beautiful places in the world. At a high alpine elevation, the campground season is short, just a five-month stretch from June (sometimes later) to mid-October. Camping here is like eating the first local strawberries of spring after a winter of tasteless hothouse fruit: intense, sweet, and fleeting. It may spoil you for anyplace else.

Saddlebag Lake is one of five intimate, nonreservable Inyo National Forest campgrounds a mere 2 miles east of the Yosemite National Park entrance station at Tioga Pass. At Tioga Lake, a cluster of open sites sprawls on the lake (but also right off CA 120). Junction Campground, at the intersection of Saddlebag Lake Road and CA 120, is a short distance off both roads but has more trees to provide privacy. Less than a mile east of Saddlebag Lake Road sits Ellery Lake, slightly downhill from CA 120. This campground has some sites well screened by shrubby willows, directly on Lee Vining Creek. Proceeding 1.6 miles up Saddlebag Lake Road, you'll find the easy-to-miss Sawmill Walk-In Campground, on the left. It's a short, level walk to a gorgeous 12-spot campground with well-spaced sites sprinkled across a rocky alpine meadow dotted with pines. At the end of Saddlebag Lake Road sits the crown jewel of the area, Saddlebag Lake, its namesake campground, and trailheads for the 20 Lakes Basin.

Saddlebag Lake is the gateway to hundreds of miles of hiking in the Hoover Wilderness.

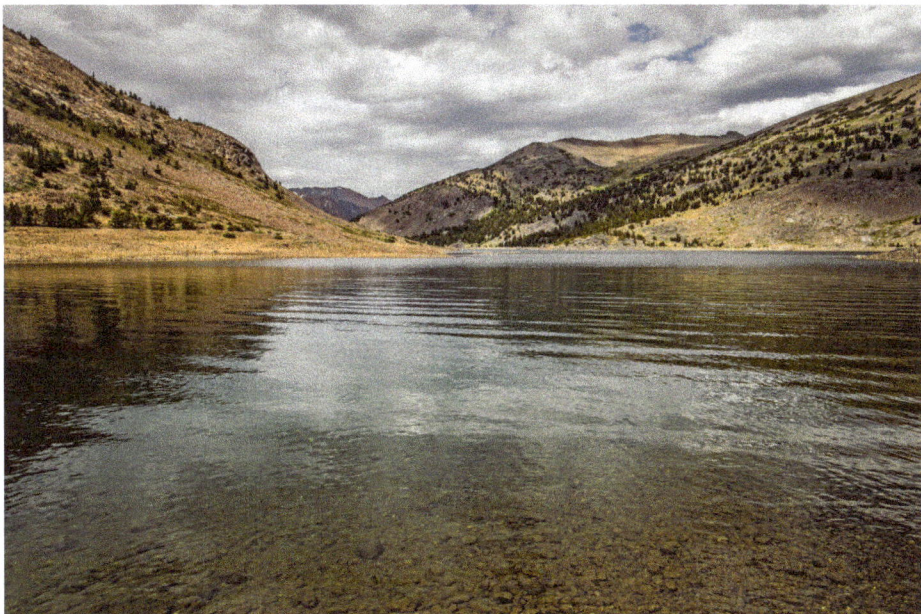

KEY INFORMATION

LOCATION: Saddlebag Lake Road, 12 miles west of I-395, Lee Vining, CA 93541

OPERATED BY: Inyo National Forest, Mono Lake Ranger District

CONTACT: Mono Basin National Forest Scenic Area Visitor Center: 760-647-3044, monolake.org/visit/vc; www.fs.usda.gov/inyo

OPEN: Mid-June–early October (weather permitting); if planning early- or late-season camping, call to be sure the campground is open

SITES: 20 sites for tents or RVs (no designated RV spots, hookups, or dump station)

EACH SITE HAS: Picnic table, fire ring, food locker

ASSIGNMENT: First come, first served; no reservations

REGISTRATION: Self-register at the information station

AMENITIES: Drinking water, vault toilets

PARKING: At individual site

FEE: $22, $7 extra vehicle; if arriving from the west, $30 entrance fee for Yosemite National Park

ELEVATION: 10,087'

RESTRICTIONS:

PETS: Dogs are permitted; must be leashed during the day and in your tent at night

FIRES: In designated fire rings only

ALCOHOL: No restrictions

OTHER: 14-day stay limit; small RVs or short trailers only; store all food and scented items in food lockers; boat rentals at resort; 15 mph speed limit on lake

---

Saddlebag Lake Campground, on a hill above the lake, is reached via a steep gravel road. Although there is plenty of daytime activity down by the lake, the campground is exceptionally quiet. Sites radiate off a single loop, and the ground is somewhat sloped, but gravel tent pads provide level pitches. The premier sites are 16, 18, and 19, which overlook the lake, but most of the other sites offer at least partial views of the water as well as the rugged peaks to the north. Spindly lodgepole pines offer only moderate screening between sites, but everyone's looking at the lake anyway.

The lake is actually a dammed reservoir, the water from which flows into Lee Vining Creek and then down to Lee Vining, where it generates power for Southern California. From the campground it's a five-minute walk to the lake for daylong fishing and hiking adventures. Rainbow trout are stocked, but the lake also holds brook, brown, and golden trout.

The elevation here is more than 10,000 feet, and until you adjust, hiking can be a lung-busting experience. A trail departs from the day-use parking lot, heading around the east side of Saddlebag Lake, a less-than-4-mile, nearly level hike. The east leg starts out above the lake, bisecting a sloping hillside where you might see Indian paintbrush and yellow wallflower blooming in summer. Small waterfalls gush downhill into the lake, where even from the trail we could see fish swimming in the clear, sapphire-blue water. The trail gradually passes through a pocket of pines then approaches the far end of the lake. Here you can extend the 4-mile experience to an 8-mile hike past a series of spectacular alpine lakes. The trail can be hard to follow near Helen and Shamrock Lakes, but there is little elevation change to contend with. Back on the west side of Saddlebag Lake, the trail crosses streams and then slips across a talus slope of rocks shed from the mountain on the right. The journey ends near the dam; continue downhill across the creek to the road, then walk back to the left and up the campground road (the worst hill of the day).

If you need ice or other supplies, Lee Vining, 12 miles east along I-395, has a few small stores, restaurants, and gas. Arriving from the west, the best bet for gas and groceries is the Central Valley town of Oakdale. Once you begin the climb into Yosemite, there are few places to buy food, and gas prices seem to rise with the elevation. Gas is available year-round at Crane Flat and (until early October) at Tuolumne Meadows, but you'll pay a premium. You can also eat in the restaurant at the Tioga Pass Resort (on the north side of CA 120 just west of Saddlebag Lake Road) and buy ice and limited other supplies there.

The campground has food-storage lockers—use them. At 11:30 p.m. a bear walked past our tent then overturned a cooler in the adjacent campsite. The bear was run off but returned at 4 a.m. and ransacked another campsite. We lay in our tent listening to the mayhem. The camp host advised that air horns are particularly effective aids to chase off marauding bears, but the idea of an air horn blast punctuating the quiet of a campground in the middle of the night is less than appealing. For the sake of your fellow campers (and the local bears), keep your food secured in the bear box.

Saddlebag Lake Campground

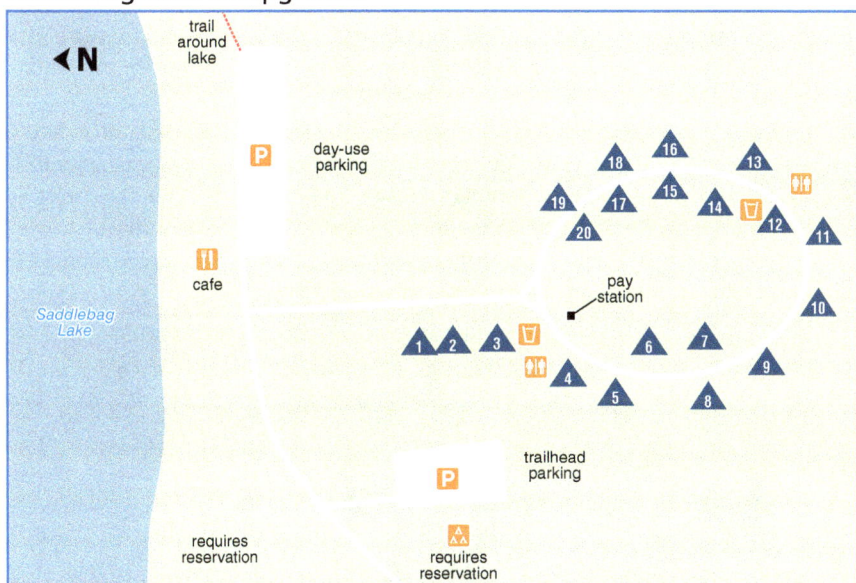

GETTING THERE

From CA 99 in Manteca, exit onto CA 120. Drive east on CA 120 through Yosemite National Park ($30 entrance fee). About 2 miles past the Tioga Pass entrance station, turn left onto Saddlebag Lake Road. Drive north 2 miles (mostly gravel), then turn right into the campground.

From US 395 in Lee Vining, go west on CA 120 about 11 miles, and turn right onto Saddlebag Lake Road. Drive north 2 miles, then turn right into the campground.

GPS COORDINATES: N37° 57.908' W119° 16.293'

50

Buckeye Campground

Beauty ★★★★★ / Privacy ★★★★★ / Spaciousness ★★★★★ / Quiet ★★★★★ / Security ★★★★★ / Cleanliness ★★★★★

Come for fishing, hiking, far-off glaciers, and the campground hot springs.

All roads that lead to Buckeye Campground also pass the Burger Barn in Bridgeport. Anytime is a good time for an everything-on-it burger, wrapped in wax paper, at the outside tables of this ageless monument to roadside dining. The historic restaurant is a famous relic of Americana. One assumes that the lean, tasty meat comes from close relatives of the sleek cattle grazing in the knee-deep grass around town. After all, this is cattle country. In Bridgeport, the heart of the Old West steadily beats.

There are four loops to the campground. The first loop you come to on the left, sites 42–68, has the campground host in site 60 (employed by WESTrek Services, the park concessionaire). Bundles of wood are sold at the host station. You continue up the hill for the other three loops.

At 7,000 feet, Buckeye is Big Country camping. The air smells of pine, dust, and cold, rushing water. Buckeye Creek runs right past the campground. The mountain wildflowers grow from the sandy, needled floor among the sage. You look up and see the rocky slopes and, farther on, the white of the glaciers on the peaks: it's cowboy country. A horse trail cuts right by the camp. The sites are mostly unoccupied, and the pitches are scoured clean by the winter. This is an excellent place to camp.

The Twin Lakes, with views of the Eastern Sierra peaks, are 4 miles from Buckeye Campground.

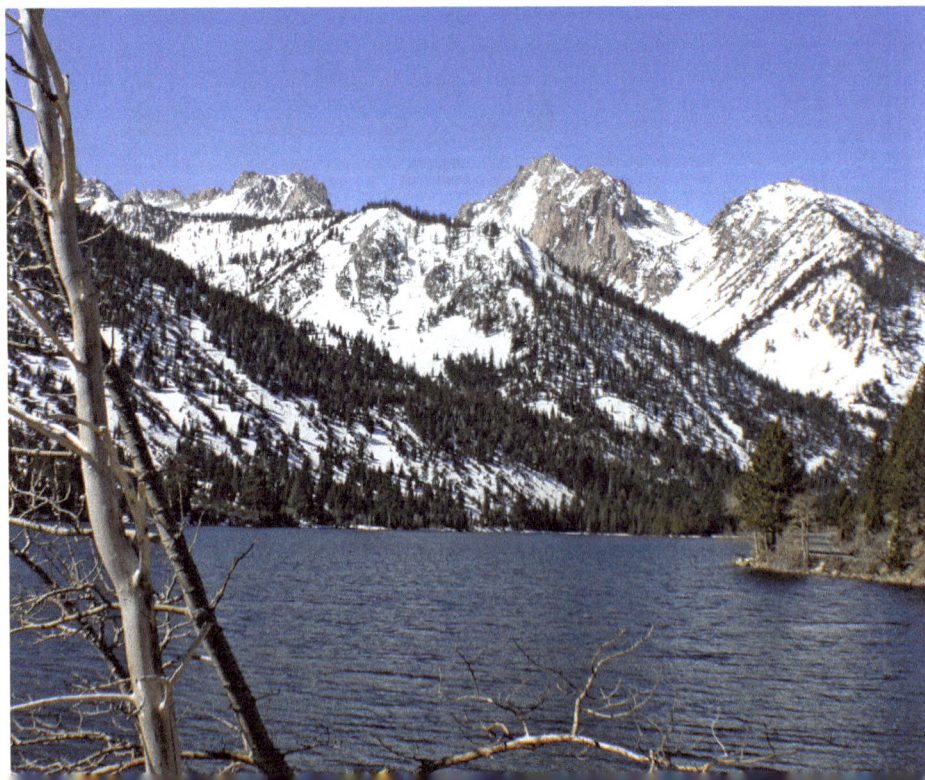

KEY INFORMATION

LOCATION: Buckeye Road, 10 miles from I-395, Bridgeport, CA 93517

OPERATED BY: Humboldt-Toiyabe National Forest, Bridgeport Ranger District

CONTACT: Bridgeport Ranger Station 760-932-7070; WESTrek Services 760-932-7092; www.fs.usda.gov/htnf

OPEN: May–early October (depending on road and weather conditions)

SITES: 67

EACH SITE HAS: Picnic table, fire ring

ASSIGNMENT: First come, first served; no reservations

REGISTRATION: At entrance to each loop

AMENITIES: Vault toilets

PARKING: At individual site

FEE: $20, $6 extra vehicle

ELEVATION: 7,500'

RESTRICTIONS:

PETS: On leash only

FIRES: In fireplace

ALCOHOL: No restrictions

VEHICLES: RVs up to 40 feet

OTHER: Don't leave food out; no potable water at campground—bring your own water

Fishing is not bad on Buckeye Creek between the two bridges—that's where the fish are stocked. You can hike over to Twin Lakes and rent a boat. Go for the big brown trout. In 1987 the state record holder, a 26.5-pounder, was caught here. However, most of the folks I saw with fish had caught little rainbows. The water-skiing on Upper Twin scares away some of the trout, so the best fishing is on Lower Twin. I talked with one old-timer who said the best time to come for the browns is in May, when it is cold and windy. Troll with Rapalas (3- to 4-inch minnows), he advised. I threw in some salmon eggs and didn't get a nibble.

Another big draw at Buckeye Campground is the hot springs. They are by the stream down from the campground. It's best to get in your car and drive down the hill. Take your first left and climb a slight hill. There is a slanting parking area immediately on the right. Climb down the steep slope to the hot pools by the river below. This can be fun. Wear shoes with some bite, as the footing is slippery. Sometimes the pools are empty, sometimes filled with fun-loving folks (clothing optional). I sat first in the hot pool then in Buckeye Creek to cool off.

Good hiking can be had right out of camp. Buckeye Campground is in a V between the two branches of Buckeye Creek. The two hikes follow the two branches upstream and ultimately swing around and join one another, so you can make up to a 16-mile loop. Bring fishing gear, as there are elusive brown trout and rainbow in the upper reaches; use local worms and try the pools behind beaver dams. The trailhead to the two hikes is up above the campground loops. Just walk up the access road (newly tarred and graveled), which will dead-end into a horse corral and the trailhead (see the map posted there).

One trail heads west along the right-hand branch of Buckeye Creek. This trail follows an erstwhile wagon road through flowered meadows and pine forest. The trail up the left branch of Buckeye Creek can be accessed from the campground's left loops (looking west). Just walk to the creek and head up the fisherman's trail. Otherwise, walk from the trailhead a few hundred yards until the trail winds left up a ridge to the stream. The wildflowers in July were all over the place—lupine, shooting star, paintbrush. Watch the campground notice board for ranger wildflower nature walks; they are fun.

Bring ice: the nearest supplies are at Doc and Al's, or Bridgeport. Think about cooling your beer and sodas in the stream. Or bring a collapsible cooler, fill it with ice, and put it in a cool place. Mind the bears. Put all your food in the car trunk when you are gone. Bears are busy tending their cubs and looking for chow during camping season. By fall, bears max out, eating 20,000 calories every day in preparation for hibernation.

Take a side trip to Bodie (bring food and water), Mono Lake, and the Virginia Creek Settlement (once part of Dogtown, a gold-rush mining camp) for a look around and a meal. Or go gem-hunting near Bridgeport: Head 3.3 miles north from Bridgeport on CA 182 and turn right on Forest Service Road 046. Head out exploring, but avoid any active mines for quartz crystals, chalcopyrite, and pyrite.

Buckeye Campground

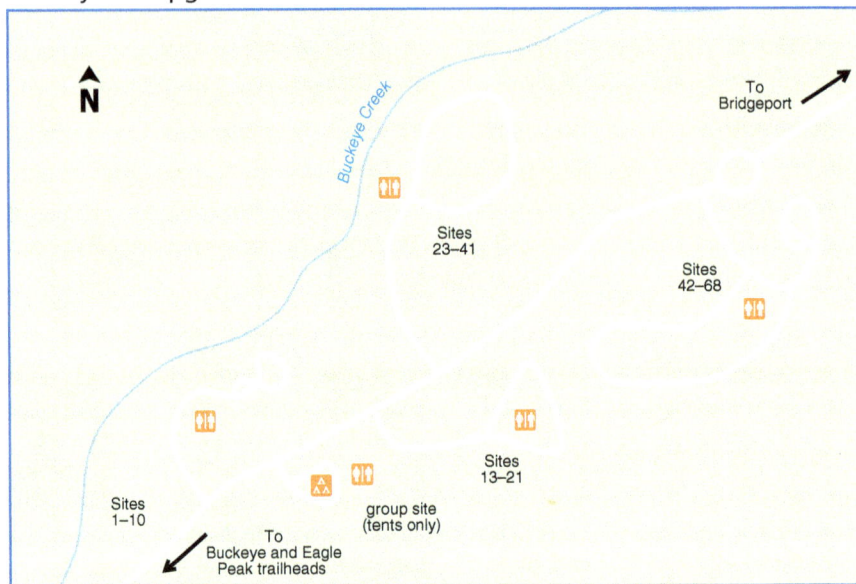

N

Buckeye Creek

To
Bridgeport

Sites
23–41

Sites
42–68

Sites
13–21

Sites
1–10

group site
(tents only)

To
Buckeye and Eagle
Peak trailheads

GETTING THERE

From Bridgeport, take Twin Lakes Road 7 miles southwest to Buckeye Road, which is on the right by Doc and Al's Resort. Go 3 miles north on Buckeye Road; veer left and continue the last mile to the campground.

GPS COORDINATES: N38° 14.268' W119° 20.767'

APPENDIX A

CAMPING-EQUIPMENT CHECKLIST

Except for the large and bulky items on this list, I keep a plastic storage container full of the essentials of car camping so that they're ready to go when I am. I make a last-minute check of the inventory, resupply anything that's low or missing, and away I go!

COOKING UTENSILS

Bottle opener
Bottles of salt, pepper, spices, sugar, cooking oil, and maple syrup in waterproof, spill-proof containers
Bowls
Can opener
Corkscrew
Cups, plastic or tin
Dish soap *(biodegradable)*, sponge, and towel
Flatware
Food of your choice
Frying pan
Fuel for stove
Matches in waterproof container
Plates
Pocketknife
Pot with lid
Spatula
Stove
Aluminum foil
Wooden spoon

FIRST AID KIT

Adhesive bandages
Antibiotic cream
Diphenhydramine *(Benadryl)*
Gauze pads
Ibuprofen or aspirin
Insect repellent
Moleskin
Snakebite kit
Sunscreen/lip balm
Tape, waterproof adhesive

SLEEPING GEAR

Pillow
Sleeping bag
Sleeping pad, inflatable or insulated
Tent with ground tarp and rainfly

MISCELLANEOUS

Bath soap *(biodegradable)*, washcloth, and towel
Camp chair
Candles
Cooler
Deck of cards
Fire starter
Flashlight or headlamp with fresh batteries
Inclement-weather clothing *(useful year-round at higher altitudes)*
Paper towels
Plastic ziplock bags
Sunglasses
Toilet paper
Water bottle
Wool blanket

OPTIONAL

Barbecue grill
Binoculars
Field guides on bird, plant, and wildlife identification
Fishing rod and tackle
Hatchet
Lantern
Maps (road, topographic, trails)

APPENDIX B

SUGGESTED READING

Alt, David D. and Donald W. Hyndman. *Roadside Geology of Northern and Central California.* Missoula, MT: Mountain Press Publishing Co., 2016.

Farquhar, Francis P. *History of the Sierra Nevada.* Oakland, CA: University of California Press, 2007.

Holliday, J. S. *The World Rushed In.* Norman, OK: University of Oklahoma Press, 2002.

Lorentzen, Bob. *The Mendocino Coast Glove Box Guide.* Mendocino, CA: Bored Feet Press, 2003.

McKinney, John. *Day Hiker's Guide to California's State Parks.* Santa Barbara, CA: Trailmaster, 2014.

Miller, Joaquin. *The Complete Poetical Works of Joaquin Miller.* Whitefish, MT: Kessinger Publishing, 2004.

Petralia, Joseph F. *Gold! Gold!* Reno, NV: Sierra Outdoor Products Co., 1996.

Rocca, Al. *Shasta Lake: Boomtowns and the Building of Shasta Dam (Images of America).* Charleston, SC: Arcadia Publishing, 2002.

Schoenherr, Allan A. *A Natural History of California.* Oakland, CA: University of California Press, 2017.

Stienstra, Tom. *California Camping.* Berkeley, CA: Moon, 2015.

———. *Northern California Camping.* Berkeley, CA: Moon, 2015.

Whitehill, Karen and Terry Whitehill. Revised by Shane Shepherd and Owen Wozniak. *Best Short Hikes in California's North Sierra.* Seattle: Mountaineers Books, 2003.

APPENDIX C

SOURCES OF INFORMATION

BENTON HOT SPRINGS
866-466-2824
760-933-2287
bentonhotsprings.org

BIG BASIN REDWOODS STATE PARK
831-338-8860
www.parks.ca.gov

BUREAU OF LAND MANAGEMENT, CALIFORNIA STATE OFFICE
916-978-4400
blm.gov/california

BUTANO STATE PARK
650-879-2040
www.parks.ca.gov

CALAVERAS BIG TREES STATE PARK
209-795-2334
www.parks.ca.gov

CALIFORNIA STATE PARKS
916-653-6995
800-777-0369
www.parks.ca.gov

DEL NORTE COAST REDWOODS STATE PARK
707-465-7335
www.parks.ca.gov

D. L. BLISS STATE PARK
530-525-7277
www.parks.ca.gov

ELDORADO NATIONAL FOREST
530-622-5061
www.fs.usda.gov/eldorado

GROVER HOT SPRINGS STATE PARK
530-694-2248
www.parks.ca.gov

HUMBOLDT REDWOODS STATE PARK
707-946-2409
www.parks.ca.gov, humboldtredwoods.org

HUMBOLDT-TOIYABE NATIONAL FOREST
775-331-6444
www.fs.usda.gov/htnf

JEDEDIAH SMITH REDWOODS STATE PARK
707-458-3294
www.parks.ca.gov

KLAMATH NATIONAL FOREST
530-842-6131
www.fs.usda.gov/klamath

LASSEN NATIONAL FOREST
530-257-2151
www.fs.usda.gov/lassen

LASSEN VOLCANIC NATIONAL PARK
530-595-4480
nps.gov/lavo

LAVA BEDS NATIONAL MONUMENT
530-667-8113
nps.gov/labe

MACKERRICHER STATE PARK
707-964-9112
www.parks.ca.gov

MCARTHUR–BURNEY FALLS MEMORIAL STATE PARK
530-335-2777
www.parks.ca.gov

MODOC NATIONAL FOREST
530-233-5811
www.fs.usda.gov/modoc

PACIFIC GAS & ELECTRIC COMPANY
916-386-5164
recreation.pge.com

PATRICK'S POINT STATE PARK
707-677-3570
www.parks.ca.gov

PLUMAS-EUREKA STATE PARK
530-836-2380
www.parks.ca.gov

PRAIRIE CREEK REDWOODS STATE PARK
707-488-2039
www.parks.ca.gov

SALT POINT STATE PARK
707-847-3221
www.parks.ca.gov

RUSSIAN GULCH STATE PARK
707-937-5804
www.parks.ca.gov

SHASTA-TRINITY NATIONAL FOREST
530-226-2500
www.fs.usda.gov/stnf

SIX RIVERS NATIONAL FOREST
707-442-1721
www.fs.usda.gov/srnf

STANISLAUS NATIONAL FOREST
209-532-3671
www.fs.usda.gov/stanislaus

SUGARLOAF RIDGE STATE PARK
707-833-5712
sugarloafpark.org

TAHOE NATIONAL FOREST
530-265-4531
www.fs.usda.gov/tahoe

VAN DAMME STATE PARK
707-937-5804
www.parks.ca.gov

U.S. FOREST SERVICE, PACIFIC SOUTHWEST REGION
707-562-8737
www.fs.usda.gov/r5

INDEX

ABOUT THE AUTHOR

WENDY SPEICHER

Wendy's love affair with the outdoors started in childhood, as she was growing up on her parents' 10-acre farm in rural Northern Michigan. Memories of nights spent in the pop-up camper in the state's sandy campgrounds and of campfire-cooked dinners of baked potatoes, corn on the cob, and sirloin steaks are still some of her fondest. Wanderlust runs deep in the family gene pool, and it drew Wendy to Northern California's Yosemite Valley on a summer break between college semesters. After that, there was no turning back.

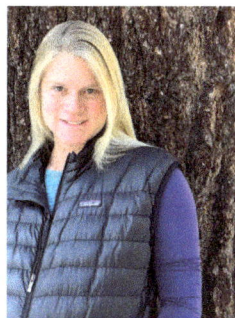
photographed by Greg Speicher

Wendy studied journalism at beautiful Humboldt State University and cut her teeth in the business covering sports, recreation, food, and entertainment at a variety of newspapers, magazines, and websites in the Lake Tahoe–Truckee and Sacramento area. Her first book, *Day & Section Hikes: Pacific Crest Trail: Northern California,* was published by Wilderness Press in 2010.

As a young mother, Wendy has temporarily retired her long-distance hiking shoes in favor of the car-camping experience, which allows her the convenience of introducing her son, Archer, to outdoor living without the burden of a fully loaded pack. Spending time outside with Archer and her husband, Greg, is the joy of her life. As a true jack-of-all-trades, when she isn't writing, Wendy is a professional massage therapist and yoga and fitness instructor and enjoys helping people attain new levels of health and well-being. Learn more at wendyspeicher.com.

DEAR CUSTOMERS AND FRIENDS,

SUPPORTING YOUR INTEREST IN OUTDOOR ADVENTURE, travel, and an active lifestyle is central to our operations, from the authors we choose to the locations we detail to the way we design our books. Menasha Ridge Press was incorporated in 1982 by a group of veteran outdoorsmen and professional outfitters. For many years now, we've specialized in creating books that benefit the outdoors enthusiast.

Almost immediately, Menasha Ridge Press earned a reputation for revolutionizing outdoors- and travel-guidebook publishing. For such activities as canoeing, kayaking, hiking, backpacking, and mountain biking, we established new standards of quality that transformed the whole genre, resulting in outdoor-recreation guides of great sophistication and solid content. Menasha Ridge Press continues to be outdoor publishing's greatest innovator.

The folks at Menasha Ridge Press are as at home on a whitewater river or mountain trail as they are editing a manuscript. The books we build for you are the best they can be, because we're responding to your needs. Plus, we use and depend on them ourselves.

We look forward to seeing you on the river or the trail. If you'd like to contact us directly, visit us at menasharidge.com. We thank you for your interest in our books and the natural world around us all.

SAFE TRAVELS,

Bob Sehlinger

BOB SEHLINGER
PUBLISHER